SENESCENCE - PHYSIOLOGY OR PATHOLOGY

Edited by **Jolanta Dorszewska**
and **Wojciech Kozubski**

Senescence - Physiology or Pathology
http://dx.doi.org/10.5772/65533
Edited by Jolanta Dorszewska and Wojciech Kozubski

Contributors

Jekaterina Erenpreisa, Kristine Salmina, Mark Steven Cragg, Jose De Jesús Serrano-Luna, Ruth Pacheco-Rivera, Jaime Arellanes-Robledo, Ruth Heinz, Sebastian Moschen, Paula Fernandez, Norma Paniego, Agustín López Gialdi, Colomba Falcone, Sara Bozzini, Jitka Rychtarikova, Klara Hulikova, Jolanta Dorszewska, Marta Kowalska, Michal Prendecki, Katarzyna Wize, Joanna Nowakowska, Michal Owecki, Michalina Maria Wężyk, Cezary Żekanowski

Published by InTech

Janeza Trdine 9, 51000 Rijeka, Croatia

Publishing Process Manager Maja Bozicevic
Technical Editor SPi Global
Cover InTech Design team

First published August, 2017
Printed in Croatia
Legal deposit, Croatia: National and University Library in Zagreb

Additional hard copies can be obtained from orders@intechopen.com

Senescence - Physiology or Pathology, Edited by Jolanta Dorszewska and Wojciech Kozubski
p. cm.
Print ISBN 978-953-51-3461-9
Online ISBN 978-953-51-3462-6

For EU product safety concerns:
IN TECH d.o.o., Prolaz Marije Krucifikse Kozulić 3, 51000 Rijeka, Croatia,
info@intechopen.com or visit our website at intechopen.com.

Meet the editors

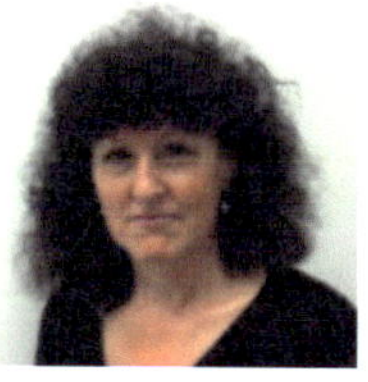

Editor, Professor Jolanta Dorszewska is Chief of Laboratory of Neurobiology, Department of Neurology, Poznan University of Medical Sciences (PUMS), Poznan, Poland. She graduated from PUMS (M.Sc. Pharmacy, 1987), obtained PhD degree at PUMS (1996) and D.Sc. in Medical Sciences at PUMS (2004). Between the years 1999 and 2000, she worked as a Research Scientist at the Institute for Basic Research in Developmental Disabilities, New York, USA. Professor Dorszewska has authored and co-authored about 100 papers (e.g. Oncotarget, Curr. Alzheimer Res., Seizure) mainly concerning the pathophysiology of Parkinson's and Alzheimer's diseases as well as epilepsy and migraine. She is a co-author and co-editor of books on genetic and biochemical factors in neurological diseases. She is a guest editor of two theme issue in Current Genomics (2014, 2013) and a member of editorial board in Advanced Alzheimer's Disease (USA).

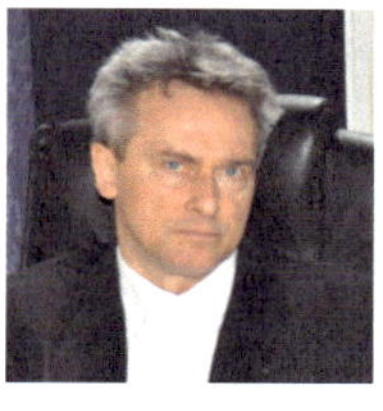

Co-Editor, Prof. Wojciech Kozubski is Head of Chair & Department of Neurology, University of Medical Sciences in Poznan, Poland. Prof. Wojciech Kozubski graduated in Medical School in Lodz, Poland, in 1980. During the years 1980–1983, he was a PhD student in the Department of Neurology, Medical School in Lodz, and next—after his PhD degree—an assistant, adjunct scientific worker and assistant professor in this department. He was scholarshiped in Academic Unit of Neuroscience of Charing Cross & Westminster Medical School, University of London (1987–1988); Department of Neurology in Sackler School of Medicine, University of Tel-Aviv (1990) and in Department of Neurology in University of Trondheim, Norway (1990–1991). Prof. Kozubski is an author and co-author of over 290 papers (102 of them are original) concerning mainly the pathophysiology of migraine and related headaches, pathophysiology of stroke, dementia, treatment of head aches and stroke. He is a co-author and co-editor of the Handbook of Clinical Neurology for neurologists, on brain tumors, affective diseases of nervous system, therapy in neurology. He is an editor of the Handbook of Treatment in Neurology and co-author and co-editor of the Hand books of Clinical Neurology for medical students. He is a co-author of the monograph on stroke aphasia. During the years 2011–2014, he was the President of Polish Neurological Society; in the years 1999–2001, President of Polish Headache Society.

Contents

Preface IX

Chapter 1 **Introductory Chapter: Molecular Basis of Senescence 1**
Jolanta Dorszewska and Wojciech Kozubski

Chapter 2 **Genetic Factors Associated with Longevity in Humans 5**
Sara Bozzini and Colomba Falcone

Chapter 3 **Sunflower Leaf Senescence: A Complex Genetic Process with Economic Impact on Crop Production 29**
Sebastián Moschen, Agustín I. López Gialdi, Norma Paniego, Paula Fernandez and Ruth Amelia Heinz

Chapter 4 **Accelerated Senescence of Cancer Stem Cells: A Failure to Thrive or a Route to Survival? 45**
Jekaterina Erenpreisa, Kristine Salmina and Mark Steven Cragg

Chapter 5 **Aging and Neurological Diseases 63**
Marta Kowalska, Michal Owecki, Michal Prendecki, Katarzyna Wize, Joanna Nowakowska, Wojciech Kozubski, Margarita Lianeri and Jolanta Dorszewska

Chapter 6 **Presenilins Interactome in Alzheimer's Disease and Pathological Ageing 95**
Michalina Maria Wężyk and Cezary Żekanowski

Chapter 7 **Is Senescence Important in Hepatic Diseases? 119**
Ruth Pacheco Rivera, Jaime Arellanes Robledo and Jesús Serrano Luna

Chapter 8 **Potential Reduction in Mortality Associated with the Shifts of Population Educational Structures in the Czech Republic 139**
Jitka Rychtaříková and Klára Hulíková Tesárková

Preface

Nowadays, the aging process is explained on the basis of ambiguous hypotheses. According to one of them, the weakening of the defenses and repair mechanisms occurs in the old organism. Another hypothesis indicates molecular changes, at the biochemical and genetic level during aging. The effect of these changes is the resistance of old cells with damaged, unrepaired DNA to the onset of apoptosis or autophagy. This leads to a higher number of diseases typical for old age such as atherosclerosis, muscular dystrophy, pulmonary disorders and other organs, neurodegenerative diseases, and many cancers.

This publication sums up the knowledge of the genetic and biochemical factors changing during senescence. We summarize the pathophysiology observed both in aging people and in the plant world. The book also contains the latest views on molecular mechanism of liver dysfunction in old age.

We hope that this book may help in understanding the complex mechanisms of senescence pathogenesis and can be an inspiration to find factors to prevent senile diseases and to treat them effectively.

Professor Jolanta Dorszewska, MD, PhD
Laboratory of Neurobiology, Department of Neurology
Poznan University of Medical Sciences
Poland

Professor Wojciech Kozubski, MD, PhD
Chair, Department of Neurology
Poznan University of Medical Sciences
Poland

Chapter 1

Introductory Chapter: Molecular Basis of Senescence

Jolanta Dorszewska and Wojciech Kozubski

Additional information is available at the end of the chapter

http://dx.doi.org/10.5772/intechopen.70214

1. Introduction

In humans, the threshold of normal aging is accepted to involve the age of 60 years. At the same time, the age above the normal aging was divided into three subgroups, including young olds (65–75 years of age), old olds (75–85 years), and eldest olds (above 85 years of age) [1]. Normal aging is defined as weakening of the repair and defense processes of the body. The weakening of the defense in aging organism leads to increase in the level of toxic factors such as reactive oxygen species (ROS), calcium ions, and immuneinflammatory response. The consequence of the change in the level of these molecular factors is the development of age-related diseases, among others, atherosclerosis, tumors and neurodegenerative diseases. Simultaneously, ROS may lead to the damage of macromolecular compounds, such as lipids, proteins, and DNA [2, 3]. ROS may also play an important role in the modulation of transcription factors activation, gene expression, and various life processes of a cell.

2. Genetic factors and normal aging

It seems that the aging process is determined by both changes in the levels of biochemical factors as well as multiple genetic variants. It is believed that normal aging is associated with genes such as *SIRT1, AKT1* and *CDKN1A*, while longevity with e.g. *FOXO3A* and *CETP*. On the other hand, weakness of cognitive function during senescence may be modified by poly-T variants of *TOMM40* and *APOE* alleles via influencing the level of apolipoprotein E [4, 5].

A detailed description of the molecular factors in aging process is provided in the chapter on genetic factors associated with longevity. According to the authors, longevity may be a complex polygenic trait influenced by many genetic changes. In addition, longevity phenomena are influenced by both epigenetic and environmental factors.

The aging process may be traced based on experimental models using candidate genes enabling early detection of aging before the emergence of typical phenotypes. Such experimental model may be plants because they allow for the examination of complex mechanisms of molecular changes during aging.

In the last years, publications point to the involvement of many molecular factors in the development of normal aging. However, we still did not prevent the pathological changes in the aging organism in the form of cardiologic, neurological, or oncological diseases.

3. Aging and old age diseases

In the aging process, functions of the p53 protein, *genome trader*, are impaired. The p53 protein does not lead to repair cells with damaged DNA or does not direct them to the path of apoptosis. The effect of these functional changes is increased susceptibility to infections, autoimmune diseases and cancers, including malignancies [1, 2]. The pathogenesis of tumors associated with the p53 protein is contained in this book.

In addition, older people often develop neurological diseases including Alzheimer's and Parkinson's diseases, epilepsy, and stroke. Based on the modern knowledge, it is difficult to separate normal and pathological aging, and neurodegeneration of central neurons. More information in the chapter, normal aging and neurodegenerative disorders.

The aging process is not limited to the central nervous system. It also includes other organs such as heart and liver. It is believed that the loss of liver regenerative capacity is disturbed in the elderly. Defective liver cells undergo apoptosis or aging. Aging cells are responsible for fibrosis and hepatocellular carcinoma. Is senescence important in hepatic diseases, available in this book.

Moreover, recently a growing interest focuses on senescent cells in the context of old age diseases, malignancy and insulin resistance, and as a therapeutic goal to prolong health.

4. Summary

Despite current intensive research on the aging process, many questions about the pathomechanism of disorders in the old body remain unanswered. Moreover, the causes of unfavorable changes in the aging organism are not fully understood. It is not known which factors precisely define aging and/or longevity and contributes to the development of senility. Finding unknown paths in the pathogenesis of aging may improve the comfort of life of elderly and protect them from diseases typical for old age.

http://dx.doi.org/10.5772/intechopen.70214

Author details

Jolanta Dorszewska[1]* and Wojciech Kozubski[2]

*Address all correspondence to: dorszewskaj@yahoo.com

1 Laboratory of Neurobiology, Department of Neurology, Poznan University of Medical Sciences, Poznan, Poland

2 Chair and Department of Neurology, Poznan University of Medical Sciences, Poznan, Poland

References

[1] Dorszewska J. Cell biology of normal brain aging: Synaptic plasticity-cell death. Aging Clinical and Experimental Research. 2013;**25**:25-34. DOI: 10.1007/s40520-013-0004-2

[2] Dorszewska J, Adamczewska-Goncerzewicz Z. Oxidative damage to DNA, p53 gene expression and p53 protein level in the process of aging in rat brain. Respiratory Physiology & Neurobiology. 2004;**139**:227-236

[3] Dorszewska J, Adamczewska-Goncerzewicz Z, Szczech J. Apoptotic proteins in the course of aging of central nervous system in the rat. Respiratory Physiology & Neurobiology. 2004;**139**:145-155

[4] Prendecki M, Florczak-Wyspiańska J, Kowalska M, Lianeri M, Kozubski W, Dorszewska J. Normal aging and dementia. In: Moretti DV, editor. Update on Dementia. Rijeka: InTech; 2016. pp. 251-272

[5] Dorszewska J, Prendecki M, Oczkowska A, Dezor M, Kozubski W. Molecular basis of familial and sporadic Alzheimer's disease. Current Alzheimer Research. 2016;**13**:952-963

Chapter 2

Genetic Factors Associated with Longevity in Humans

Sara Bozzini and Colomba Falcone

Additional information is available at the end of the chapter

http://dx.doi.org/10.5772/intechopen.69637

Abstract

Introduction: Life expectancy and the rate of survival into old age have risen dramatically throughout the past century. The positive ageing outcomes may be due to a variety of factors including healthy lifestyle behaviors, but it is clear that longevity has a genetic basis, with heritability estimate of 20–35%. In this contest, it was emerged that human longevity seems strongly influenced by gender defined as the combination between biological sexual characteristics and factors related to behavior, social role, lifestyle and life experiences. Body—research methods: Successful ageing seems to be related to gene involved in different pathways of regulation, such as immune-inflammatory responses and oxidative stress. The aims of the present review are to discuss recent findings and highlight the genetic basis of longevity. For these reasons we are aimed to describe the most important underpinning which is the gender differences in longevity between males and females. Conclusion—key results: It appears clear that longevity may represent a complex polygenic trait that is influenced by the interaction of multiple genetic variants, as was demonstrated by several genetic studies conducted in the last years. Furthermore, epigenetic and environmental factors actin on the longevity phenotype.

Keywords: longevity, genetic basis, healthy lifestyle, inflammation, oxidative stress, epigenetics

1. Introduction

Human life expectancy has increased over the last two centuries worldwide [data shown by the World Health Organization, 2012], and this is mainly due to improvement of health care, lifestyle and nutrition. Considering the continuous increase of lifespan and the consequent growth of the elderly population, research on ageing has been continuously increasing in the last decades. The age threshold used to define "longevity" varies by study but is typically ≥ 85 years old and "exceptional longevity" may be considered at age ≥ 95 years old [1].

Many epidemiological data conducted in different populations indicate the presence of a strong familial component of longevity. These studies demonstrate that parents, siblings and offspring of long-lived subjects have significant survival advantage. In particular, it seems that these subjects had higher probability to become long-lived persons and to have a lower risk to undergo the most important age-related diseases, such as cardiovascular diseases (CVD), diabetes and cancer. For these reasons, most of the human ageing studies concentrate around long-lived families, including highly and middle-aged members.

The presence of strong familial component of longevity led to hypothesize the presence of a genetic basis, most likely expected to be polygenic, and was demonstrated a heritability estimates of 20–35% [2]. In fact, human lifespan is a complex trait which is assumed to be determined by many genes with small individual effects [3].

The gerontogenes, genes controlling ageing and longevity, are highly interconnected and related to stress response [4]. Prolonged or severe stress exposure exhausts the defence mechanism accelerating the process of ageing by accumulation of mistakes and physiological abnormalities. Nevertheless, on the other hand, it is known that moderate stress could have beneficial effects stimulating innate defence resources of the body thereby by expression of gene responsible for stress resistance. This stimulation increases the body ability to cope with higher levels of stress and slows down ageing in the so-called lifespan hormesis effect [5].

Genomic studies into ageing thus far focus on the determinants of human lifespan variation by using age at death, prospective survival, disease-free survival or exceptional longevity as outcome. From a genomic perspective, individuals from long-lived families are assumed to be characterized by a decreased prevalence of disease-promoting variants and an increased prevalence of variants conferring maintenance of health and protection from disease, when compared to population controls [6]. However, in 2010 a study conducted by Beekman et al. [7] tested whether a set of alleles increase the risk of coronary artery disease, cancer and type 2 diabetes for compatibility with human longevity, but they found that longevity is not compromised by the cumulative effect of this set of risk alleles for common disease.

Studies in the field of genetics aim to decipher the impact of variation in the DNA structure that either can be inherited and are therefore found in the germ line DNA or that arises during an individual's lifespan. Core end points in the field of genetics are (1) single nucleotide polymorphisms (SNPs), which are single base variations in the DNA structure which are found in 1% of the population or more and (2) copy number variations, which are segments of DNA that vary in copy number between genomes of different individuals ranging from one kilobase to several megabases in size.

Genome-wide association study (GWAS) of human longevity has accumulated lots of data. In order to provide insight into the process of ageing, the applications of integrative genomic may to evaluate heritability of transcripts and identify sequence polymorphism can be useful. Very few copy number variations (CNVs) have been found to be linked with successful ageing and remain the area of active investigation in immune-related genes involved in ageing. A comprehensive consciousness of the interactions between genetic factors involved in the regulation of immune system will help know their roles in longevity and age-related diseases. They also will provide guidance for personalized efforts to intervene in the ageing process.

During ageing, vital bodily function, such as regeneration and reproduction slowly declines and the loss of essential body function leads to age-related pathologies, which ultimately cause death [8]. A large part of ageing phenotype is explained by an imbalance between inflammatory and anti-inflammatory response, which result in "inflammaging", a low-grade chronic pro-inflammatory status of ageing. Successful ageing seems to be related to pointing out that polymorphisms for the immune system genes, which are involved in the regulation of immune-inflammatory responses, may play a key role in the genetics of ageing. Another important pathway implicated in longevity concerns the oxidative stress. The balance between pro-oxidants and enzymatic antioxidant systems may be of particular importance in the elderly. In this scenario, nutritional deficiencies and sedentary lifestyle concur with a depletion of dietary antioxidants and increased susceptibility to oxidative stress.

Women live longer than men, and this difference in life expectancy is a worldwide phenomenon indicating that human longevity seems strongly influenced by gender defined as the combination between biological sexual characteristics and factors related to behavior, social role, lifestyle and life experiences [9].

The aims of the present review are to discuss recent findings, highlight the genetic basis of longevity and describe the most important underpinning which is the gender differences in longevity between males and females.

2. Insulin-like signaling pathway

The most studied pathway that regulates the ageing process is the insulin-like pathways. Briefly, upon insulin-like growth factor-1 (IGF-1) binding to IGF-1 receptor (IGF-1R), the intracellular phosphoinositol-3-kinase (PI3K) is activated, leading to formation of the downstream intermediate phosphoinositide-3,4,5-trisphosphate. The latter binds to 3-phosphoinositide-dependent kinase 1 (PDK-1), which, in turn, phosphorylates and activates the kinases Akt/PKB and *s*erum- and *g*lucocorticoid-inducible *k*inase (*SGK-1*) that control regular growth processes in the cell. Together, the stress resistance factors, among which forkhead box gene, group O (FOXO) transcriptional factor, are activated [10]. This signaling activity is reduced in long-lived subjects of different species, such as nematode, mice and humans.

Gene encoding for protein involved in this pathway contains mutation correlated to longevity. In particular, mutation in IGF-1R gene in humans was associated to longer survival compared to usual [11]. Furthermore, in animal models, mutation in genes encoding for substrates of insulin receptors 1 and 2 results in the extended lifespan [12], and mutations in genes encoding kinases PI3K, AKT/PKB and PDK are associated with a prolonged life [13].

Insulin-like signaling inhibits the mechanisms of stress response regulated by FOXO transcription factor [14]. In mammals, there are four FOXOs (FOXO1, FOXO3, FOXO4, FOXO6) that regulate different genes in different cell types [15]: FOXO3 may undergo a greater decline with ageing. The mechanism by which longevity-associated alleles of FOXO3 reduce age-related mortality is currently of great clinical interest. FOXO3 has been associated with longevity in multiple candidate gene association studies in diverse groups including German, Italian and Chinese centenarians [16–18]. The precise mechanism by which FOXO3A influences longevity may be due to its effects on oxidative stress, insulin sensitivity and cell cycle progression [2]. A recent GWAS meta-analysis observed only a modest association of FOXO3 with survival to ≥90 years of age [6]. Further, in a genome-wide linkage analysis among nonagenarians, linkage to FOXO3 and another forkhead box gene, FOXO1, was not detected [19]. The lack of an association observed in these studies may be due to small sample sizes of exceptionally long-lived individuals, as the association of FOXO3 with longevity is stronger in persons aged ≥ 95 years and especially in centenarians [17, 18].

3. Lipid metabolism

Lipid metabolism is downregulated with time, leading to age-dependent diseases, such as metabolic syndrome and atherosclerosis. As previously demonstrated, dyslipidemia is associated with altered activity in a number of genes.

Three major genes of lipid metabolism are involved longevity, the genes encoding for apolipoprotein E (APOE), cholesteryl ester transfer protein (CETP) and peroxisome proliferator-activated receptor (PPAR).

In prior candidate gene association, variants of APOE have been consistently associated with longevity. The APOE gene encoded for the apolipoprotein E, a protein that combines with lipids in the body to form lipoproteins, and are responsible for packaging cholesterol and other fats and carrying them through the bloodstream. Maintaining normal levels of cholesterol is essential for the prevention of disorders that affect the heart and blood vessels (CVD), including heart attack and stroke, and consequently it contributed to good ageing.

The APOE gene has three common polymorphic alleles, leading to six possible genotypes [20], called ε2, ε3 and ε4. The most common allele is ε3, which is found in more than half of the general population. Both ε4 and ε2 alleles have been associated with cardiovascular disease (CVD) risk [21]. The associations with CVD may be related to the involvement of these isoforms in inflammation, elevated lipid levels and oxidative stress [22]. Some studies have observed that APOE2 occurs at a higher frequency in the elderly and centenarians, suggesting an association with longevity [23]; on the contrary, APOE4 may be less common in these groups and associated with early mortality [24]. However, a study conducted in Italian subjects showed that the ε2 allele is associated with an increased likelihood of longevity. Interestingly, all of the Italian centenarians of the study were free of cognitive impairment and major age-related diseases, suggesting an association of ε2 allele with successful ageing [25].

A particular chromosomal region, 19q13.11–q13.32 showed linkage with longevity, as shown in a large genome-wide linkage scan among nonagenarian sibling pairs of the European ancestry [19]; subsequent association analyses using GWAS data found that APOE4 and APOE2 alleles explain linkage at this region. Further studies are needed to elucidate the role of rare APOE variants on longevity and healthy ageing.

Variants in the CETP gene, which is involved in the regulation of high-density lipoprotein levels, were previously suggested as markers of exceptional longevity and healthy ageing in Ashkenazi Jews and Japanese-American men, respectively [26, 27]. However, in a recent case-control study among Han Chinese long-lived individuals, none of the four SNPs in the promoter region of the CETP gene was associated with longevity [28]. Additionally, a meta-analysis of eight studies did not observe an association between CETP polymorphisms and longevity [29].

Peroxisome proliferator-activated receptors (PPARs) are ligand-inducible transcription factors that belong to the nuclear hormone receptor superfamily. PPAR ligands comprise fatty acids and their derivatives. PPARα is activated by fatty acids, eicosanoids, 15-d prostaglandin and oxidized fatty acids. PPARα function antagonizes the metabolic syndrome and ageing in general [30], through regulation of genes promoting lipid oxidation and metabolism of lipoproteins, such as main apolipoprotein of high density, Apo A-1.

4. Inflammation

Inflammation forms the basis of many physiological and pathological processes. Much is known about how inflammation is initiated, develops and resolves over the short term. But less is known about the causes and consequences of chronic inflammation. Chronic inflammation, by contrast, is a prolonged, dysregulated and maladaptive response that involves active inflammation, tissue destruction and attempts at tissue repair. Such persistent inflammation is associated with many chronic human conditions and diseases, including allergy, atherosclerosis, cancer, arthritis and autoimmune diseases [31].

A large part of the ageing phenotype is explained by an imbalance between inflammatory and anti-inflammatory networks, which results in the low-grade chronic pro-inflammatory status of ageing, called "inflammaging" [32], which appears accelerated in many age-associated diseases. The source of the age-associated chronic inflammation was mainly attributed to the progressive activation of immune cells over time and to the acquisition of a specific senescent cell phenotype [33]. Thus, the accumulation of senescent cells in aged subjects could contribute to the perpetuation of "inflammaging", and the systemic chronic inflammatory status could, in turn, contribute to the disease development.

Data on case-control studies suggest that the presence of pro-inflammatory genotype is unfavorable for the achievement of extreme longevity in good health and, in addition, it likely favors the onset of age-related diseases, such as CVD and Alzheimer's disease, major causes of mortality and disability in the elderly. In the contrary, it was shown that centenarians have an increased level of inflammatory mediators in comparison to old subjects, but they also have a high level of anti-inflammatory cytokines together with protective genotypes.

Genes implicated in inflammatory pathways may be associated with longevity, as was demonstrated in a case-control study in which a homozygous genotype of the RAGE gene was more frequently found in male long-lived subjects [34]. A study in German long-lived cases and younger controls observed that cases were less likely to be deficient in complement C4 long genes, suggesting a potential role of immunity in lifespan [35].

The cellular communication has a fundamental role in regulating the reaction of the immune system to a possible danger [36]. In this scenario, a key role may be played by Toll-like receptor 4 (TLR4) that initiated both innate and clonotypic immunity to Gram-negative bacteria and to other agents. A SNP in TLR4 gene, ASP299GLY, was known to regulate the receptor signaling that the presence of 896G allele seems to be attenuated with a minor risk to develop carotid atherosclerosis and less intima-media thickness in the common carotid artery. In addition, 896G TLR4 allele shows a significantly lower frequency in patients affected by acute myocardial infarction with respect to controls, whereas centenarians show higher frequency [37]. This is in agreement with the hypothesis that genetic basis of inflammation might play an opposite role in CVD and in longevity because people genetically predisposed to a weak inflammatory activity less likely develop CVD and, at the same time, without any serious infectious disease complication, more likely live longer [38].

TLR4 activates the inflammatory cell via the NF-kB pathway by inducing the expression of a variety of cytokines; some of these have been shown to be involved in atherosclerosis and reciprocally in longevity. In a previous study, conducted by Candore et al. [39], it was demonstrated that the 896 G allele carriers produce low levels of the pro-inflammatory cytokines IL-6 and tumor necrosis factor (TNF)-α and a higher level of the anti-inflammatory cytokine IL-10.

Cytokines are the expression of a network involving genes, polymorphisms and environment, and are involved both in inflammation and anti-inflammation. Pro-inflammatory cytokines seem to play a pathogenic role in age-related diseases, and in previous study, it was demonstrated that genetic variations located within their promoter regions may influence the susceptibility to age-related diseases, by increasing gene transcription and therefore cytokine production [40, 41]. Conversely, successful ageing seems to be associated to genetic variations determining increased production of anti-inflammatory cytokines or decreased production of pro-inflammatory cytokines, suggesting a role for the control of the inflammatory state in the attainment of longevity.

IL-1, IL-2, IL-6, IL-12, IL-15, IL-18, IL-22, IL-23, TNF-α and interferon (IFN)-γ were described as pro-inflammatory cytokines, while IL-1Ra, IL-4, IL-10 and TGF-β1 as anti-inflammatory cytokines. High levels of IL-1, together with IL-6, tumor necrosis factor (TNF) and interferon (IFN)-γ, are associated with increased risk of morbidity and mortality in the older subject. Two studies have investigated the role of genetic variability of IL-1 gene cluster and a possible association with longevity [42, 43]. Neither study showed statistically significant differences comparing the allele frequencies, genotype frequencies and haplotype frequencies between long-lived patients and youth nor between males or females.

Also, IL-6 cytokine polymorphisms have been linked to longevity. Several data suggest that IL-6 −174C/G locus variability seems to modulate individual susceptibility to common causes of morbidity and mortality among the oldest subjects (e.g. type 2 diabetes, CVD and dementia) and therefore interferes with an individual's ability to reach the extreme limits of human lifespan [44–47]. A meta-analysis, conducted in Europeans, analyzed that data regarding long-lived subjects and controls from eight case-control studies showed no association between the IL-6 polymorphism and the probability of achieving a very old age. However, in Italian centenarians the IL-6 −174GG genotype appeared to be negatively associated with longevity and reduced the chance for male GG carriers of achieving centenarian status [48]. Also, a Turkish study, conducted by Kayaaltı et al. [49], found an association between IL-6 −174G/C promoter region polymorphism and longevity.

As regards TNF polymorphisms, it was found that there was no association between distribution of TNF-α −308 genotypes and longevity [43, 50]. However, GA genotype was associated with decreased prevalence of dementia in centenarians, and, in centenarians, the AA genotype was associated to higher mortality risk and higher plasma levels of TNF-α [51].

Studies evaluating IFN-γ polymorphisms in longevity showed no association [52, 53]. A gender study evaluated the distribution of +874T → A IFN-γ polymorphisms in 174 Italian centenarians and showed that +874T allele was found less frequently in centenarian women than in centenarian men or in control women, whereas no significant differences were observed in the distribution of the two alleles between male and female controls. These data seem to strengthen the idea that gender may be a major variable in the biology of the ageing process [54].

According to the best of our knowledge, there is no data in the literature to support significant associations between polymorphisms in the anti-inflammatory cytokines and longevity.

Accumulated data strongly suggest that besides chronic up-regulation of pro-inflammatory genes and cytokines, also cyclooxygenases are induced during the ageing process. In fact, cyclooxygenases (COX-1 and COX-2), key enzymes in the conversion of arachidonic acid to the precursors of bioactive lipid mediators, prostaglandin, thromboxane and prostacyclin, and lipoxygenases (LOX) enzymes that catalyze the stereospecific insertion of molecular oxygen into various positions in arachidonic acid, were intimately involved in inflammation. Previous studies have shown that −765GC and −1708GA SNPs in the promoter region of COX-2 gene and 5-LOX genes, respectively, resulting in a significant lower promoter activity, were found to be associated with reduced risk of severe atherosclerosis [55]. In centenarians the frequencies of these pro-inflammatory alleles were significantly lower, whereas age-related controls were higher [56].

Ageing and longevity are complex traits resulting not only and not exclusively from genetics but rather from the interactions between genetics, environment and chance.

5. Oxidative stress

The role of the oxidative stress response in healthy ageing and longevity is a hot topic in the field of human ageing studies.

The free radical theory of ageing, proposed in 1956, suggests that free radical-induced accumulation of damage to cellular macromolecules is a primary driving force of ageing and a major determinant of lifespan [57]. Under normal conditions ROS (including NADPH oxidases (NOX), mitochondria, xanthine oxidase, monoamine oxidase and nitric oxide synthase) were maintained at the physiological levels by several endogenous antioxidant systems, such as superoxide dismutatase (SOD), catalase, glutathione peroxidases and glutathione reductase (GR). Other antioxidant systems involving thiol-disulfide oxidoreductase systems include the cytosolic proteins thioredoxin (TRX) and glutaredoxin (GRX). ROS at physiological levels can interact with redox state and play a role in mediating cell signaling, while at pathological levels can result in oxidative damage to cellular components that activate several cell death pathways.

The close interrelationship of redox balance to oxidative stress has in recent years become a more prominent aspect of the free radical theory of ageing that was extended to implicate the mitochondrial production of ROS [58]. In fact, studies in long-lived species showed the presence of reduced oxidative damage [59], reduced mitochondrial free radical production [60], increased antioxidant defences [60] and increased resistance to oxidative stress both in vivo and in vitro [61]. However, a lack of correlation of oxidation with lifespan [62], or even an increase in oxidative damage/stress associated with long lifespan, has also been reported [63].

In addition, in support of the importance of genetic factors in the ageing organism's ability to counteract the negative effects of oxidative stress, genetic modifications of the stress response with age have also been reported. These modifications may minimize health risks, and they may increase the individual's possibilities of achieving a longer life [64].

Several studies suggest that both genetic factors and modifiable lifestyle habits have major impact on the oxidative stress response, but the relative contribution of genes and lifestyle in promoting an efficient stress response in cells is difficult to estimate. Data collected in the literature shows that in experimental organisms and in exceptionally long-lived individuals, among the antioxidant enzymes, a major role in longevity seems to be attributed to genes SOD2 and GPX [65].

Knowing that oxidative stress accelerates telomere loss, the genes encoding the telomere maintenance pathway, mainly telomerase reverse transcriptase (TERT) and telomerase RNA component (TERC), are also important to happen [66, 67]. In addition, in support of gender difference in longevity, some genes involved in the stress response pathway, like heat shock protein A1A (HSPA1A) or paraoxonase 1 (PON1), show sex-specific effects [68].

A study in Chinese centenarians and nonagenarians and younger controls identified significant genotype differences in the GNB3 and eNOS genes, whose variants have been implicated in hypertension and vascular function via nitric oxide (NO) generation, respectively [69]. Another study found that variants of two NO synthase genes, NOS1 and NOS2, decrease the probability of attaining longevity, suggesting that NO production and signaling may be involved in ageing [70].

Mitochondrial genetic variability, both germ line and somatic, influences the stress response and is associated with human ageing/longevity. In both physiological and pathological conditions, a strict coordination between nuclear and mitochondrial genomes is necessary to ensure the biosynthesis and functional activity of mitochondria [71]. In normal conditions, signals from the nucleus to mitochondrion are essential for maintaining an adequate mitochondrial structure and function. The mitochondrial replication and transcription were modulated by several nuclear-encoded transcription factors and coactivators, such as transcription factors which bind to the promoter regions of mtDNA (transcription factors A (Tfam) and B (mtTFB) that enhancing the rate of transcription initiation of mtDNA genes and mitochondrial biogenesis) and nuclear respiratory factors NRF-1 and NRF-2 and the peroxisome proliferator-activated receptor-γ coactivator-1 (PGC-1) family coactivators (PGC-1α, PGC-1α,and related coactivator PRC) [71–73].

Although many association studies explored the effect of genetic variability at candidate genes belonging to the oxidative stress pathway in relation to age-related clinical conditions [74], as well as with human longevity, few papers investigated their role on the quality of human ageing and in particular on the functional decline characterizing human senescence. Most of the studies investigate the association of genes related to oxidative stress with cognitive ability and cognitive ageing in healthy older people [75–79] and found an involvement of apolipoprotein E (APOE), catechol-O-methyltransferase (COMT), brain-derived neurotrophic factor (BDNF) and dystrobrevin-binding protein 1 (DTNBP1) genes in cognitive ability in older people.

A recent work conducted by Dato et al. [80] investigated the association between 311 SNPs at 38 genes belonging to the oxidative stress pathway with functional status at very older age. They found associations for TXNRD1 variability with activities of daily living and walking speed, NDUFS1 and UCP3 with handgrip strength and walking speed and GCLC and UCP2 with walking speed. They also found that the association between genetic variability in the pro-oxidant-antioxidant pathway and functional status at old age is influenced by sex and in particular in nonagenarian females. From these data it is possible to speculate that pro-oxidant-antioxidant pathway is able to modulate physical and cognitive performance after the ninth decade of life, finally influencing extreme survival.

Thus, the balance between pro-oxidants and enzymatic antioxidant systems may be of particular importance in the elderly, whose nutritional deficiencies and sedentary lifestyle concur with a depletion of dietary antioxidants and increased susceptibility to oxidative stress.

6. Gender and longevity

The impact of gender difference in ageing has been extensively assessed, but the precise mechanisms of interaction between a series of fundamental aspects, such as hormonal, immunological and metabolic pathways as well as genetic background remain largely unknown. The high prevalence of women among centenarians suggests that men and women follow different trajectories to reach extreme longevity. In particular, females benefited from healthier lifestyles and favorable environmental conditions in the past century [81]. Moreover, the differences in longevity between genders are related to free radical production because mitochondrial oxidative stress is higher in males than females. Estrogens in women confer better protection against ageing, through an up-regulated expression of antioxidant longevity-related genes [82]. In support of this, there are also some available epidemiologies of age-related diseases confirming substantially different between genders and showing changes dramatically in women after menopause [83].

Much research has been carried out into the role of sex hormones in determining lifespan [84], and one hypothesis is that sex hormones appear to influence the immune system. It is well known that estrogens, androgens and progesterone affect cells of the innate and adaptive immune system differently during the reproductive phase of life [85]. It is widely recognized that estrogens inhibit natural killer cell cytotoxicity and reduce neutrophil chemotaxis and consequently inflammation [86, 87]. Moreover, macrophages treated in vitro with oestradiol display a reduced production of pro-inflammatory cytokines, such as IL-1β, IL-6 and TNF-α [88]. Estrogens and androgens are responsible for a reduced immature number of T-lymphocytes and thymus involution after puberty [89] and can also influence the adaptive immunity in an opposing way, contributing to an improved humoral response in women but also favoring the appearance of autoreactive clones and the susceptibility to autoimmune diseases [90].

The sudden loss of ovarian estrogen and progesterone production that characterizes menopause induces pathophysiological changes in different organs and systems [91], bone density, breast cellular composition, cardiovascular health, mood/cognitive function and sexual well-being. Menopause reflects the inevitable final hallmark of a woman's fertile lifespan and of the above-described beneficial effects of estrogens on immune responses. Rapid reduction of estrogen levels results in an increased susceptibility and mortality toward a series of infectious diseases caused in old women losing of their immunological privilege toward infection [85, 92].

It is noteworthy that women will soon spend half of their life in postmenopause, if the current trend of increasing human life expectancy should persist.

7. Lifestyle and physical activity

The ageing process is dynamic and characterized by a continuous remodeling, and it appears evident that the main actors are DNA repair, apoptosis, immune response, oxidative stress and inflammation that these mechanisms are necessary to interact in an efficient way. But life expectancy at birth has been increasing in western societies thanks to the continuous improvement of medical assistance with respect to age-related diseases, especially CVD and cancer, environmental factors and lifestyle.

Among lifestyle factors, having a major impact on the whole organism oxidative stress response, there are impaired nutrition, reduced physical activity, alcohol consumption and cigarette smoking, which are major contributors to the failure of systemic homeostasis, especially if persisting for a long part of the individual's life. For these reasons the effects of physical activity and diet in oxidative stress response in humans have been suggested that both are able to tip the balance of oxidative burden/antioxidant response.

In support of this hypothesis, it has been reported that dietary restricted mice, which live much longer and show a very delayed aging phenotype [93, 94]. Thus, dietary restriction can trigger a molecular genetic response which postpones ageing and age-related phenotypes. Specifically, reduced glucose metabolisms result in an increase in ROS accumulation by stimulating the basal metabolic rate and consequently increase oxidative stress [95]. This has brought to search for drugs or interventions which may act on these mechanisms without the side effects of calorie restriction [96]. Among the most important measures in this context, you may name the protein restriction and the use of drugs involved in the IGF-1 axis and in the FOXO/TOR pathway [97]. As emerged from the analysis of data resulting from studies in geographical areas with exceptional longevity (such as Sardinia and Okinawan), it seems to be important to follow a low-protein diet, such as the Mediterranean diet [98]. In these cases, the traditional diet seems to allow to stimulate molecular mechanisms that increase the lifespan. The Mediterranean diet and red wine consumption, rich in antioxidants like resveratrol, have been shown to have protective effects against oxidative damage. People who consume large amounts of fruits and vegetables have a lower incidence of CVD, stroke and tumors, and it has been proposed that the assumption of micro-nourishments with antioxidant activity could be responsible for the reduction of chronic diseases [99]. Consistently, long-lived individuals seem to prefer a diet rich in vegetables and in natural antioxidants. In addition, lower degree of oxidative stress was found in healthy Okinawan centenarians compared to aged subjects, data obtained by measuring the level of lipid peroxide and tocopherol (Vitamin E) in plasma [100]. Okinawan diet, with its high intake of green leafy and yellow-root vegetables, sweet potatoes as a dietary staple and soy as a principle protein, supplemented by small amounts of fish and meat, may be a significant advantage in achieving their exceptionally long life expectancy, thanks to a particularly high amount of antioxidant vitamins [102]. However, this finding could be due not only to nutritional factors [101] but also to a specific genetic background.

Moderate physical activity attenuates several age-related diseases, reduces blood pressure in hypertensive patients [103] and improves the serum lipid profile with an average reduction of 3.7% in triglyceride and 5% in low-density lipoprotein (LDL)-cholesterol levels and a 4.6% increase of HDL-cholesterol levels [104]. Benefits derived by physical activity in older people, for the maintenance of an optimal health status and the prevention or management of chronic diseases, can derive from exercise-induced adaptations of the cellular antioxidant defence systems [105]. In these subjects indeed, the presence of higher serum levels of antioxidants associated with higher strength and physical performance was demonstrated [106, 107].

8. Epigenetics

In the field of longevity, more recent studies have shown that an important role is also played by epigenetics. In fact, studies in various models have revealed that genetic differences and somatic modulations underlie longevity, but also non-genetic factors play an important role. These considerations have pointed out the importance of epigenetic mechanisms in modulating longevity pathways.

Epigenome, the intermediate layer of genomic information between the genome and transcriptome, is another molecular level that could provide additional insight in the processes of ageing. Epigenetic regulation of transcription is mediated by histone modification, DNA methylation and microRNAs.

Chromatin and epigenetic factors influenced gene expression dynamically by regulating access of transcriptional machinery to DNA. It is clear that, with age, there is a general loss of histones coupled with local and global chromatin remodeling, an imbalance of activating and repressive histone modifications and transcriptional change in all ageing models.

Additionally, particularly in mammalian systems, there is a global and local change in DNA methylation, site-specific loss and gain in heterochromatin and significant nuclear reorganization

Methylation patterns of genes involved in, for example, development and morphogenesis, DNA binding and regulation of transcription [108, 109], seem to change with age; a progressive linear increase in methylation with age at the ELOVL2 gene was found in a cohort of 501 long-lived individuals [110].

The epigenomic field recently became more accessible for the screening of large study populations; however, larger studies, new methodologies and the consistent use of different study designs to follow up results might help to unravel the genomic component of healthy ageing and longevity.

It was proposed that a mathematical model, on the basis of the methylation levels of 353 CpG units, formulated a mathematical model, the so-called epigenetic clock, which was able to predict the chronological age of a subject starting from the methylation level of several cells and tissues of his body [111]. This model also indicates that methylation represents one of the most accurate biomarkers of age and it was able to predict all-cause mortality also after adjusting for traditional risk factors [112]. Finally, when it was used to estimate the biological age of several tissues from supercentenarians, it has been demonstrated that the brain and muscle represent the youngest tissues of these exceptional individuals [113].

However, even if the relationship between methylation process and ageing is still not clear, this discovery has some wide potential applications, ranging from detailed monitoring of changes occurring with age to forensic purposes. It therefore appears clear that future advances in this field could help the understanding of the complex physiology of ageing, lifespan and age-associated diseases.

Starting from the observations, epigenetic modifications affect not only the ageing process but also its quality [114]. Epigenome-wide association studies identified hundreds of sites spread along the entire genome in which methylation levels change between the oldest old and younger subjects.

Although serum microRNAs play roles in the diagnosis of various diseases, little is known about circulating miRNAs in the ageing process. Human serum from healthy individuals contains abundant quantities and species of circulating miRNAs, and they can be readily detected with almost all routine RNA analysis techniques, including qRT-PCR. Zhang et al. evaluated miRNA expression profiles in the sera of healthy individuals at different steps of the ageing process, and they found a different miRNA regulation in the ageing process. In particular, they found that miRNAs changed significantly in the ageing process: miR-29b, miR-106b, miR-130b, miR-142-5p and miR-340 decreased, and miR-92a, miR-222 and miR-375 increased [115].

Evidence provided suggested also that TLR signaling transduction is impaired in cells from aged animals, as suggested by lack of response to the stimulation of lipopolysaccharide (LPS), and the increased pro-inflammatory cytokine release observed in macrophages of aged mice even if no conclusive results can be obtained on the TLR baseline expression level in animal model during ageing [116]. In particular, a trio of miRNA, such as miR-155, miR-21 and miR-146a, has proven to be key TLR signaling modulators, and, importantly, these miRNAs are codified by endotoxin-responsive genes [117].

9. Discussion

Human longevity is an extremely complex trait on which genetic, epigenetic and environmental factors act. It is becoming evident that the genetic differences concur lowly to life expectancy before 60 years, but their impact on survival becomes more prominent at old ages. Unfortunately, the currently available knowledge is not sufficient to explain the secret of longevity, even because available data, reviewed in this work, are sometimes conflicting. The precise reason for these data discrepancy is unknown; however, several factors may be involved, such as ethnic, lifestyle and cultural differences among the population analyzed in the diverse studies.

During the past decade, several longevity gene candidates have been identified; the majority of them concern components of the inflammatory system, stress response or lipid and glucose metabolism.

As discussed above, longevity is characterized by a balance between pro-inflammatory and anti-inflammatory agents, which act as key players. A pro-inflammatory propensity can confer high resistance against infectious diseases, but it also may increase susceptibility to inflammation-based diseases. On the other hand, an anti-inflammatory tendency, instead, may cause an increased susceptibility to infections and might not allow to reach a more advanced age. According to a perspective suggested in recent years, the best candidates to become centenarians are not the strongest, and most robust subjects among their age cohort, but subjects that better adapt to the environment, show more biological plasticity.

Since genetic variants may exert small to moderate effects on human longevity, additional prospective investigation with large sample size is needed to elucidate the role of genetic variation. It may also be worthwhile for future studies to evaluate the genetic basis of ageing separately in male and female, which is especially importantly given the longer lifespan of females.

Therefore, the balance between lifestyle and physiological changes during ageing on the one hand and risk factors for age-associated diseases on the other should be taken into consideration. Several studies suggest that on the oxidative stress response both genetic factors and modifiable lifestyle have major impact. Studies in experimental organisms and in exceptionally long-lived individuals have tried to identify genetic factors modulating the oxidative stress response, but the relative contribution of genes and lifestyle in promoting an efficient stress response in cells is difficult to estimate.

Data deriving from different studies indicate that stress response pathway is an integrated network of molecular activities, ranging from immunity to inflammatory regulation and activation, to glucose homeostasis and mitochondrial metabolism. Therefore, ageing seems to be associated with a loss of complexity in the dynamics of multiple control systems that may reduce the ability to adapt to stress, leading to a state of impaired homeostasis and vulnerability to internal and external stressors. On the contrary, the healthy oldest old seems be able to maintain a higher level of integration among the different physiological pathways operating within the cell, thus interacting more successfully with stressors.

Author details

Sara Bozzini[1]* and Colomba Falcone[1,2,3]

*Address all correspondence to: sara-84@tiscali.it

1 Interdepartimental Centre for Research in Molecular Medicine (CIRMC), University of Pavia, Pavia, Italy

2 Department of Cardiology, Istituti Clinici di Pavia e Vigevano University Hospital, Pavia, Italy

3 IRCCS San Donato Hospital, San Donato Milanese, Italy

References

[1] Rajpathak SN, Liu Y, Ben-David O, Reddy S, Atzmon G, Crandall J, Barzilai N. Lifestyle factors of people with exceptional longevity. Journal of the American Geriatrics Society. 2011 Aug;**59**(8):1509-1512. DOI: 10.1111/j.1532-5415.2011.03498.x

[2] Newman AB, Murabito JM. The epidemiology of longevity and exceptional survival. Epidemiologic Reviews. 2013;**35**:181-197. DOI: 10.1093/epirev/mxs013

[3] Finch CE, Tanzi RE. Genetics of aging. Science. 1997 Oct 17;**278**(5337):407-411

[4] Moskalev AA. Evolutionary ideas on the nature of aging. Advances in Gerontology. 2011;**1**:112-121. DOI: 10.1134/S207905701102010X

[5] Cornelius C, Perrotta R, Graziano A, Calabrese EJ, Calabrese V. Stress responses, vitagenes and hormesis as critical determinants in aging and longevity: Mitochondria as a "chi". Immunity and Ageing. 2013;**10**:15. DOI: 10.1186/1742-4933-10-15

[6] Deelen J, Beekman M, Uh HW, Broer L, Ayers KL, Tan Q, Kamatani Y, Bennet AM, Tamm R, Trompet S, Guðbjartsson DF, Flachsbart F, Rose G, Viktorin A, Fischer K, Nygaard M, Cordell HJ, Crocco P, van den Akker EB, Böhringer S, Helmer Q, Nelson CP, Saunders GI, Alver M, Andersen-Ranberg K, Breen ME, van der Breggen R, Caliebe A, Capri M, Cevenini E, Collerton JC, Dato S, Davies K, Ford I, Gampe J, Garagnani P, de Geus EJ, Harrow J,

van Heemst D, Heijmans BT, Heinsen FA, Hottenga JJ, Hofman A, Jeune B, Jonsson PV, Lathrop M, Lechner D, Martin-Ruiz C, Mcnerlan SE, Mihailov E, Montesanto A, Mooijaart SP, Murphy A, Nohr EA, Paternoster L, Postmus I, Rivadeneira F, Ross OA, Salvioli S, Sattar N, Schreiber S, Stefánsson H, Stott DJ, Tiemeier H, Uitterlinden AG, Westendorp RG, Willemsen G, Samani NJ, Galan P, Sørensen TI, Boomsma DI, Jukema JW, Rea IM, Passarino G, de Craen AJ, Christensen K, Nebel A, Stefánsson K, Metspalu A, Magnusson P, Blanché H, Christiansen L, Kirkwood TB, van Duijn CM, Franceschi C, Houwing-Duistermaat JJ, Slagboom PE. Genome-wide association meta-analysis of human longevity identifies a novel locus conferring survival beyond 90 years of age. Human Molecular Genetics. 2014 Aug 15;**23**(16):4420-4432. DOI: 10.1093/hmg/ddu139

[7] Beekman M, Nederstigt C, Suchiman HE, Kremer D, van der Breggen R, Lakenberg N, Alemayehu WG, de Craen AJ, Westendorp RG, Boomsma DI, de Geus EJ, Houwing-Duistermaat JJ, Heijmans BT, Slagboom PE. Genome-wide association study (GWAS)-identified disease risk alleles do not compromise human longevity. Proceedings of the National Academy of Sciences of the United States of America. 2010 Oct 19;**107**(42):18046-18049. DOI: 10.1073/pnas.1003540107

[8] Moskalev AA, Pasyukova EG. From theories of aging to anti-aging interventions. Frontiers in Genetics. 2014 Aug 14;**5**:276. DOI: 10.3389/fgene.2014.00276

[9] Regitz-Zagrosek V. Sex and gender differences in health. Science & Society Series on Sex and Science. EMBO Reports. 2012 Jun 29;**13**(7):596-603. DOI: 10.1038/embor.2012.87

[10] Hartl FU. Cellular homeostasis and aging. Annual Review of Biochemistry. 2016 Jun 2;**85**:1-4. DOI: 10.1146/annurev-biochem-011116-110806

[11] Suh Y, Atzmon G, Cho MO, Hwang D, Liu B, Leahy DJ, Barzilai N, Cohen P. Functionally significant insulin-like growth factor I receptor mutations in centenarians. Proceedings of the National Academy of Sciences of the United States of America. 2008;**105**:3438-3442. DOI: 10.1073/pnas.0705467105

[12] Selman C, Lingard S, Choudhury AI, Batterham RL, Claret M, Clements M, Ramadani F, Okkenhaug K, Schuster E, Blanc E, et al. Evidence for lifespan extension and delayed age-related biomarkers in insulin receptor substrate 1 null mice. The FASEB Journal. 2008;**22**:807-818. DOI: 10.1096/fj.07-9261com

[13] Narasimhan SD, Yen K, Tissenbaum HA. Converging pathways in lifespan regulation. Current Biology. 2009;**19**:R657–R666. DOI: 10.1016/j.cub.2009.06.013

[14] Morris BJ, Willcox DC, Donlon TA, Willcox BJ. FOXO3: A major gene for human longevity—A mini-review. Gerontology. 2015;**61**(6):515-525. DOI: 10.1159/000375235

[15] Paik JH, Kollipara R, Chu G, Ji H, Xiao Y, Ding Z, Miao L, Tothova Z, Horner JW, Carrasco DR, Jiang S, Gilliland DG, Chin L, Wong WH, Castrillon DH, DePinho RA. FoxOs are lineage-restricted redundant tumor suppressors and regulate endothelial cell homeostasis. Cell. 2007 Jan 26;**128**(2):309-323. DOI: 10.1016/j.cell.2006.12.029

[16] Anselmi CV, Malovini A, Roncarati R, Novelli V, Villa F, Condorelli G, Bellazzi R, Puca AA. Association of the FOXO3A locus with extreme longevity in a southern Italian centenarian study. Rejuvenation Research. 2009 Apr;**12**(2):95-104. DOI: 10.1089/rej.2008.0827

[17] Flachsbart F, Caliebe A, Kleindorp R, Blanché H, von Eller-Eberstein H, Nikolaus S, Schreiber S, Nebel A. Association of FOXO3A variation with human longevity confirmed in German centenarians. Proceedings of the National Academy of Sciences of the United States of America. 2009 Feb 24;**106**(8):2700-2705. DOI: 10.1073/pnas.0809594106

[18] Willcox BJ, Donlon TA, He Q, Chen R, Grove JS, Yano K, Masaki KH, Willcox DC, Rodriguez B, Curb JD. FOXO3A genotype is strongly associated with human longevity. Proceedings of the National Academy of Sciences of the United States of America. 2008 Sep 16;**105**(37):13987-13992. DOI: 10.1073/pnas.0801030105

[19] Beekman M, Blanché H, Perola M, Hervonen A, Bezrukov V, Sikora E, Flachsbart F, Christiansen L, De Craen AJ, Kirkwood TB, Rea IM, Poulain M, Robine JM, Valensin S, Stazi MA, Passarino G, Deiana L, Gonos ES, Paternoster L, Sørensen TI, Tan Q, Helmer Q, van den Akker EB, Deelen J, Martella F, Cordell HJ, Ayers KL, Vaupel JW, Törnwall O, Johnson TE, Schreiber S, Lathrop M, Skytthe A, Westendorp RG, Christensen K, Gampe J, Nebel A, Houwing-Duistermaat JJ, Slagboom PE, Franceschi C; GEHA consortium. Genome-wide linkage analysis for human longevity: Genetics of Healthy Aging Study. Aging Cell. 2013 Apr;**12**(2):184-193. DOI: 10.1111/acel.12039

[20] Liu CC, Kanekiyo T, Xu H, Bu G. Apolipoprotein E and Alzheimer disease: Risk, mechanisms and therapy. Nature Reviews Neurology. 2013 Feb;**9**(2):106-118. DOI: 10.1038/nrneurol.2012.263. Erratum in: Nature Reviews Neurology. 2013. DOI: 10.1038/nmeurol.2013.32

[21] Lahoz C, Schaefer EJ, Cupples LA, Wilson PW, Levy D, Osgood D, Parpos S, Pedro-Botet J, Daly JA, Ordovas JM. Apolipoprotein E genotype and cardiovascular disease in the Framingham Heart Study. Atherosclerosis. 2001 Feb 15;**154**(3):529-537. DOI: 10.1016/S0021-9150(00)00570-0

[22] Jofre-Monseny L, Minihane AM, Rimbach G. Impact of apoE genotype on oxidative stress, inflammation and disease risk. Molecular Nutrition & Food Research. 2008 Jan;**52**(1):131-145. DOI: 10.1002/mnfr.200700322

[23] Seripa D, Franceschi M, Matera MG, Panza F, Kehoe PG, Gravina C, Orsitto G, Solfrizzi V, Di Minno G, Dallapiccola B, Pilotto A. Sex differences in the association of apolipoprotein E and angiotensin-converting enzyme gene polymorphisms with healthy aging and longevity: A population-based study from Southern Italy. The Journals of Gerontology. Series A, Biological Sciences and Medical Sciences. 2006 Sep;**61**(9):918-923. DOI: 10.1093/gerona/61.9.918

[24] Jacobsen R, Martinussen T, Christiansen L, Jeune B, Andersen-Ranberg K, Vaupel JW, Christensen K. Increased effect of the ApoE gene on survival at advanced age in healthy and long-lived Danes: Two nationwide cohort studies. Aging Cell. 2010 Dec;**9**(6):1004-1009. DOI: 10.1111/j.1474-9726.2010.00626.x

[25] Panza F, Frisardi V, Seripa D, Pilotto A, Solfrizzi V. Plasma levels of n-3 polyunsaturated fatty acids and cognitive decline: Possible role of depressive symptoms and apolipoprotein E genotyping. Journal of the American Geriatrics Society. 2010 Nov;**58**(11):2249-2251. DOI: 10.1111/j.1532-5415.2010.03110.x

[26] Koropatnick TA, Kimbell J, Chen R, Grove JS, Donlon TA, Masaki KH, Rodriguez BL, Willcox BJ, Yano K, Curb JD. A prospective study of high-density lipoprotein cholesterol, cholesteryl ester transfer protein gene variants, and healthy aging in very old Japanese-American men. Journal of Gerontology A Biological Science Medical Science. 2008 Nov;**63**(11):1235-1240. DOI: doi.org/10.1093/gerona/63.11.1235

[27] Barzilai N, Atzmon G, Schechter C, Schaefer EJ, Cupples AL, Lipton R, Cheng S, Shuldiner AR. Unique lipoprotein phenotype and genotype associated with exceptional longevity. JAMA. 2003 Oct 15;**290**(15):2030-2040. DOI: 10.1001/jama.290.15.2030

[28] Yang JK, Gong YY, Xie L, Yang Y, Xu LY, Zhang YP. Association study of promoter polymorphisms in the CETP gene with longevity in the Han Chinese population. Molecular Biology Reports. 2014 Jan;**41**(1):325-329. DOI: 10.1007/s11033-013-2865-z

[29] Li Q, Huang P, He QC, Lin QZ, Wu J, Yin RX. Association between the CETP polymorphisms and the risk of Alzheimer's disease, carotid atherosclerosis, longevity, and the efficacy of statin therapy. Neurobiology of Aging. 2014 Jun;**35**(6):1513.e13-23. DOI: 10.1016/j.neurobiolaging.2013.12.032

[30] Schiff M, Bénit P, Jacobs HT, Vockley J, Rustin P. Therapies in inborn errors of oxidative metabolism. Trends in Endocrinology and Metabolism. 2012;**23**:488-495. DOI: 10.1016/j.tem.2012.04.006

[31] Weiss U. Inflammation. Nature. 2008 Jul 24;**454**(7203):427. DOI: 10.1038/454427a

[32] Oliviero F, Sfriso P, Scanu A, Fiocco U, Spinella P, Punzi L. Epigallocatechin-3-gallate reduces inflammation induced by calcium pyrophosphate crystals in vitro. Frontiers in Pharmacology. 2013 Apr 17;**4**:51. DOI: 10.3389/fphar.2013.00051

[33] Campisi J. Cellular senescence and lung function during aging. Yin and Yang. Annals of the American Thoracic Society. 2016 Dec;**13**(Supplement_5):S402–S406. DOI: 10.1513/AnnalsATS.201609-703AW

[34] Falcone C, Bozzini S, Colonna A, Matrone B, Paganini EM, Falcone R, Pelissero G. Possible role of -374T/A polymorphism of RAGE gene in longevity. International Journal of Molecular Sciences. 2013 Nov 21;**14**(11):23203-23211. DOI: 10.3390/ijms141123203

[35] Flachsbart F, Caliebe A, Heinsen FA, Hemming-Karlsen T, Schreiber S, Franke A, Nebel A. Investigation of complement component C4 copy number variation in human longevity. PloS One. 2014 Jan 22;**9**(1):e86188. DOI: 10.1371/journal.pone.0086188

[36] Capri M, Salvioli S, Sevini F, Valensin S, Celani L, Monti D, Pawelec G, De Benedictis G, Gonos ES, Franceschi C. The genetics of human longevity. Annals of the New York Academy of Sciences. 2006 May;**1067**:252-263. Review. DOI: 10.1196/annals.1354.033

[37] Balistreri CR, Candore G, Colonna-Romano G, Lio D, Caruso M, Hoffmann E, Franceschi C, Caruso C. Role of Toll-like receptor 4 in acute myocardial infarction and longevity. JAMA. 2004 Nov 17;**292**(19):2339-2340. DOI: 10.1001/jama.292.19.2339

[38] Vasto S, Candore G, Balistreri CR, Caruso M, Colonna-Romano G, Grimaldi MP, Listi F, Nuzzo D, Lio D, Caruso C. Inflammatory networks in ageing, age-related diseases and longevity. Mechanisms of Ageing and Development. 2007 Jan;**128**(1):83-91

[39] Candore G, Aquino A, Balistreri CR, Bulati M, Di Carlo D, Grimaldi MP, Listì F, Orlando V, Vasto S, Caruso M, Colonna-Romano G, Lio D, Caruso C. Inflammation, longevity, and cardiovascular diseases: Role of polymorphisms of TLR4. Annals of the New York Academy of Sciences. 2006 May;**1067**:282-287. DOI: 10.1196/annals.1354.037

[40] Pawelec G, Ouyang Q, Colonna-Romano G, Candore G, Lio D, Caruso C. Is human immunosenescence clinically relevant? Looking for 'immunological risk phenotypes'. Trends in Immunology. 2002 Jul;**23**(7):330-332

[41] Bidwell JL, Wood NA, Morse HR, Olomolaiye OO, Keen LJ, Laundy GJ. Human cytokine gene nucleotide sequence alignments: Supplement 1. European Journal of Immunogenetics. 1999 Apr–Jun;**26**(2-3):135-223

[42] Cavallone L, Bonafè M, Olivieri F, Cardelli M, Marchegiani F, Giovagnetti S, Di Stasio G, Giampieri C, Mugianesi E, Stecconi R, Sciacca F, Grimaldi LM, De Benedictis G, Lio D, Caruso C, Franceschi C. The role of IL-1 gene cluster in longevity: A study in Italian population. Mechanisms of Ageing and Development. 2003 Apr; **124**(4):533-538

[43] Wang XY, Hurme M, Jylhä M, Hervonen A. Lack of association between human longevity and polymorphisms of IL-1 cluster, IL-6, IL-10 and TNF-alpha genes in Finnish nonagenarians. Mechanisms of Ageing and Development. 2001 Dec;**123**(1):29-38

[44] Antonicelli R, Olivieri F, Cavallone L, Spazzafumo L, Bonafè M, Marchegiani F, Cardelli M, Galeazzi R, Giovagnetti S, Perna GP, Franceschi C. Tumor necrosis factor-alpha gene -308G>A polymorphism is associated with ST-elevation myocardial infarction and with high plasma levels of biochemical ischemia markers. Coronary Artery Disease. 2005 Dec;**16**(8):489-493

[45] Pola R, Gaetani E, Flex A, Aloi F, Papaleo P, Gerardino L, De Martini D, Flore R, Pola P, Bernabei R. 174 G/C interleukin-6 gene polymorphism and increased risk of multi-infarct dementia: A case-control study. Experimental Gerontology. 2002 Jul;**37**(7):949-955

[46] Tonet AC, Karnikowski M, Moraes CF, Gomes L, Karnikowski MG, Córdova C, Nóbrega OT. Association between the -174 G/C promoter polymorphism of the interleukin-6 gene and cardiovascular disease risk factors in Brazilian older women. Braz J Med Biol Res. 2008 Jan;**41**(1):47-53

[47] Nigam P, Kwa S, Velu V, Amara RR. Loss of IL-17-producing CD8 T cells during late chronic stage of pathogenic simian immunodeficiency virus infection. Journal of Immunology. 2011 Jan 15;**186**(2):745-753. DOI: 10.4049/jimmunol.1002807

[48] Di Bona D, Vasto S, Capurso C, Christiansen L, Deiana L, Franceschi C, Hurme M, Mocchegiani E, Rea M, Lio D, Candore G, Caruso C. Effect of interleukin-6 polymorphisms on human longevity: a systematic review and meta-analysis. Ageing Research Reviews. 2009 Jan;**8**(1):36-42. DOI: 10.1016/j.arr.2008.09.001

[49] Kayaaltı Z, Sahiner L, Durakoğlugil ME, Söylemezoğlu T. Distributions of interleukin-6 (IL-6) promoter and metallothionein 2A (MT2A) core promoter region gene polymorphisms and their associations with aging in Turkish population. Archives of Gerontology and Geriatrics. 2011 Nov-Dec;**53**(3):354-358. DOI: 10.1016/j.archger.2011.01.001

[50] Ross OA, Curran MD, Rea IM, Hyland P, Duggan O, Barnett CR, Annett K, Patterson C, Barnett YA, Middleton D. HLA haplotypes and TNF polymorphism do not associate with longevity in the Irish. Mechanisms of Ageing and Development. 2003 Apr;**124**(4):563-567

[51] Bruunsgaard H, Benfield TL, Andersen-Ranberg K, Hjelmborg JV, Pedersen AN, Schroll M, Pedersen BK, Jeune B. The tumor necrosis factor alpha -308G>A polymorphism is associated with dementia in the oldest old. Journal of the American Geriatrics Society. 2004 Aug;**52**(8):1361-1366. DOI: 10.1111/j.1532-5415.2004.52369.x

[52] Ross OA, Curran MD, Meenagh A, Williams F, Barnett YA, Middleton D, Rea IM. Study of age-association with cytokine gene polymorphisms in an aged Irish population. Mechanisms of Ageing and Development. 2003 Feb;**124**(2):199-206

[53] Pes GM, Lio D, Carru C, Deiana L, Baggio G, Franceschi C, Ferrucci L, Oliveri F, Scola L, Crivello A, Candore G, Colonna-Romano G, Caruso C. Association between longevity and cytokine gene polymorphisms. A study in Sardinian centenarians. Aging Clinical and Experimental Research. 2004 Jun;**16**(3):244-248

[54] Lio D, Scola L, Crivello A, Bonafè M, Franceschi C, Olivieri F, Colonna-Romano G, Candore G, Caruso C. Allele frequencies of +874T-->A single nucleotide polymorphism at the first intron of interferon-gamma gene in a group of Italian centenarians. Experimental Gerontology. 2002 Jan-Mar;**37**(2-3):315-319

[55] Cipollone F, Fazia ML. COX-2 and atherosclerosis. Journal of Cardiovascular Pharmacology. 2006;**47**(Suppl 1):S26–S36

[56] Vasto S, Caruso C. Immunity & Ageing: A new journal looking at ageing from an immunological point of view. Immunity & Ageing. 2004 Oct 29;**1**(1):1. DOI: 10.1186/1742-4933-1-1

[57] Harman D. Aging: A theory based on free radical and radiation chemistry. Journal of Gerontology. 1956 Jul;**11**:298-300

[58] Harman D. The biologic clock: The mitochondria? Journal of the American Geriatrics Society. 1972 Apr;**20**(4):145-147

[59] Finkel T, Holbrook NJ. Oxidants, oxidative stress and the biology of ageing. Nature. 2000 Nov 9;**408**(6809):239-247. Review. DOI: 10.1038/35041687

[60] Pamplona R. Mitochondrial DNA damage and animal longevity: Insights from comparative studies. Journal of Aging Research. 2011 Mar 2;**2011**:807108. DOI: 10.4061/2011/807108

[61] Kregel KC, Zhang HJ. An integrated view of oxidative stress in aging: Basic mechanisms, functional effects, and pathological considerations. American Journal of Physiology. Regulatory, Integrative and Comparative Physiology. 2007 Jan;**292**(1):R18–R36. Review. DOI: 10.1152/ajpregu.00327.2006

[62] Pérez VI, Bokov A, Van Remmen H, Mele J, Ran Q, Ikeno Y, Richardson A. Is the oxidative stress theory of aging dead? Biochimica et Biophysica Acta. 2009 Oct;**1790**(10):1005-1014. DOI: 10.1016/j.bbagen.2009.06.003. Review

[63] Anson RM, Bohr VA. Mitochondria, oxidative DNA damage, and aging. Journal of the American Aging Association. 2000 Oct;**23**(4):199-218. DOI: 10.1007/s11357-000-0020-y

[64] Dato S, Crocco O, D'acquila P, Francesco de R, Bellizzi D, Rose G, Passarino G. Exploring the role of genetic variability and lifestyle in oxidative stress response for healthy aging and longevity. International Journal of Molecular Science. 2013, **14**, 16443-16472; DOI: 10.3390/ijms140816443

[65] Crawford A, Fassett RG, Geraghty DP, Kunde DA, Ball MJ, Robertson IK, Coombes JS. Relationships between single nucleotide polymorphisms of antioxidant enzymes and disease. Gene. 2012 Jun 15;**501**(2):89-103. DOI: 10.1016/j.gene.2012.04.011. Review

[66] Soerensen M, Thinggaard M, Nygaard M, Dato S, Tan Q, Hjelmborg J, Andersen-Ranberg K, Stevnsner T, Bohr VA, Kimura M, Aviv A, Christensen K, Christiansen L. Genetic variation in TERT and TERC and human leukocyte telomere length and longevity: A cross-sectional and longitudinal analysis. Aging Cell. 2012 Apr;**11**(2):223-227. DOI: 10.1111/j.1474-9726.2011.00775.x

[67] Atzmon G, Cho M, Cawthon RM, Budagov T, Katz M, Yang X, Siegel G, Bergman A, Huffman DM, Schechter CB, Wright WE, Shay JW, Barzilai N, Govindaraju DR, Suh Y. Evolution in health and medicine Sackler colloquium: Genetic variation in human telomerase is associated with telomere length in Ashkenazi centenarians. Proceedings of the National Academy of Sciences of the United States of America. 2010 Jan 26;**107**(Suppl 1): 1710-1717. DOI: 10.1073/pnas.0906191106

[68] Passarino G, Montesanto A, Dato S, Giordano S, Domma F, Mari V, Feraco E, De Benedictis G. Sex and age specificity of susceptibility genes modulating survival at old age. Human Heredity. 2006;**62**(4):213-220. DOI: 10.1159/000097305

[69] Nijiati M, Saidaming A, Qiao J, Cheng Z, Qiu C, Sun Y. GNB3, eNOS, and mitochondrial DNA polymorphisms correlate to natural longevity in a Xinjiang Uygur population. PloS One. 2013 Dec 20;**8**(12):e81806. DOI: 10.1371/journal.pone.0081806

[70] Montesanto A, Crocco P, Tallaro F, Pisani F, Mazzei B, Mari V, Corsonello A, Lattanzio F, Passarino G, Rose G. Common polymorphisms in nitric oxide synthase (NOS) genes influence quality of aging and longevity in humans. Biogerontology. 2013 Apr;**14**(2):177-186. DOI: 10.1007/s10522-013-9421-z

[71] Garesse R, Vallejo CG. Animal mitochondrial biogenesis and function: A regulatory cross-talk between two genomes. Gene. 2001 Jan 24;**263**(1-2):1-16. Review

[72] Piantadosi CA, Suliman HB. Redox regulation of mitochondrial biogenesis. Free Radical Biology & Medicine. 2012 Dec 1;**53**(11):2043-2053. DOI: 10.1016/j.freeradbiomed.2012.09.014. Review

[73] Yoboue ED, Devin A. Reactive oxygen species-mediated control of mitochondrial biogenesis. International Journal of Cell Biology. 2012;**2012**:403870. DOI: 10.1155/2012/403870

[74] Rawford A, Fassett RG, Coombes JS, Kunde DA, Ahuja KD, Robertson IK, Ball MJ, Geraghty DP. Relationship between antioxidant enzyme genotype and activity and kidney function: A case-control study. Clinical Nephrology. 2012 Aug;**78**(2):135-144. DOI: 10.5414/CN107421

[75] Deary IJ, Wright AF, Harris SE, Whalley LJ, Starr JM. Searching for genetic influences on normal cognitive ageing. Trends in Cognitive Sciences. 2004 Apr;**8**(4):178-184. DOI: 10.1016/j.tics.2004.02.008

[76] Arris SE, Deary IJ. The genetics of cognitive ability and cognitive ageing in healthy older people. Trends in Cognitive Sciences. 2011 Sep;**15**(9):388-394. DOI: 10.1016/j.tics.2011.07.004

[77] Harris SE, Fox H, Wright AF, Hayward C, Starr JM, Whalley LJ, Deary IJ. A genetic association analysis of cognitive ability and cognitive ageing using 325 markers for 109 genes associated with oxidative stress or cognition. BMC Genetics. 2007 Jul 2;**8**:43. DOI: 10.1186/1471-2156-8-43

[78] Kachiwala SJ, Harris SE, Wright AF, Hayward C, Starr JM, Whalley LJ, Deary IJ. Genetic influences on oxidative stress and their association with normal cognitive ageing. Neuroscience Letters. 2005 Sep 30;**386**(2):116-120. DOI: 10.1016/j.neulet.2005.05.067

[79] Starr JM, Fox H, Harris SE, Deary IJ, Whalley LJ. GSTz1 genotype and cognitive ability. Psychiatric Genetics. 2008 Aug;**18**(4):211-212. DOI:10.1097/YPG.0b013e328304dea8

[80] Dato S, Soerensen M, Lagani V, Montesanto A, Passarino G, Christensen K, Tan Q, Christiansen L. Contribution of genetic polymorphisms on functional status at very old age: A gene-based analysis of 38 genes (311 SNPs) in the oxidative stress pathway. Experimental Gerontology. 2014 Apr;**52**:23-29. DOI: 10.1016/j.exger.2014.01.014

[81] Franceschi C, Motta L, Valensin S, Rapisarda R, Franzone A, Berardelli M, Motta M, Monti D, Bonafè M, Ferrucci L, Deiana L, Pes GM, Carru C, Desole MS, Barbi C, Sartoni G, Gemelli C, Lescai F, Olivieri F, Marchegiani F, Cardelli M, Cavallone L, Gueresi P, Cossarizza A, Troiano L, Pini G, Sansoni P, Passeri G, Lisa R, Spazzafumo L, Amadio L, Giunta S, Stecconi R, Morresi R, Viticchi C, Mattace R, De Benedictis G, Baggio G. Do men and women follow different trajectories to reach extreme longevity? Italian Multicenter Study on Centenarians (IMUSCE). Aging (Milano). 2000 Apr;**12**(2):77-84. Review

[82] Vina J, Gambini J, Lopez-Grueso R, Abdelaziz KM, Jove M, Borras C. Females live longer than males: Role of oxidative stress. Current Pharmaceutical Design. 2011 Dec 1; **17**(36):3959-3965. Review

[83] Austad SN, Bartke A. Sex differences in longevity and in responses to anti-aging interventions: A mini-review. Gerontology. 2015;**62**(1):40-46. DOI: 10.1159/000381472

[84] Viña J, Borrás C, Gambini J, Sastre J, Pallardó FV. Why females live longer than males: Control of longevity by sex hormones. Science of Aging Knowledge Environment. 2005 Jun 8;**2005**(23):pe17. Review. DOI: 10.1126/sageke.2005.23.pe17

[85] Giefing-Kröll C, Berger P, Lepperdinger G, Grubeck-Loebenstein B. How sex and age affect immune responses, susceptibility to infections, and response to vaccination. Aging Cell. 2015 Jun;**14**(3):309-321. DOI: 10.1111/acel.12326. Review

[86] Hao S, Zhao J, Zhou J, Zhao S, Hu Y, Hou Y. Modulation of 17beta-estradiol on the number and cytotoxicity of NK cells in vivo related to MCM and activating receptors. International Immunopharmacology. 2007 Dec 15;**7**(13):1765-1775. DOI: 10.1016/j.intimp.2007.09.017

[87] Ashcroft GS, Greenwell-Wild T, Horan MA, Wahl SM, Ferguson MW. Topical estrogen accelerates cutaneous wound healing in aged humans associated with an altered inflammatory response. American Journal of Pathology. 1999 Oct;**155**(4):1137-1146. DOI: 10.1016/S0002 9440(10)65217-0

[88] Kramer PR, Kramer SF, Guan G. 17 beta-estradiol regulates cytokine release through modulation of CD16 expression in monocytes and monocyte-derived macrophages. Arthritis and Rheumatism. 2004 Jun;**50**(6):1967-1975. DOI: 10.1002/art.20309

[89] Olsen NJ, Kovacs WJ. Evidence that androgens modulate human thymic T cell output. Journal of Investigative Medicine. 2011 Jan;**59**(1):32-35

[90] Sakiani S, Olsen NJ, Kovacs WJ. Gonadal steroids and humoral immunity. Nature Reviews Endocrinology. 2013 Jan;**9**(1):56-62. DOI: 10.1038/nrendo.2012.206. Review

[91] Vrachnis N, Zygouris D, Iliodromiti Z, Daniilidis A, Valsamakis G, Kalantaridou S. Probing the impact of sex steroids and menopause-related sex steroid deprivation on modulation of immune senescence. Maturitas. 2014 Jul;**78**(3):174-178. DOI: 10.1016/j.maturitas.2014.04.014. Review

[92] Ossewaarde ME, Bots ML, Verbeek AL, Peeters PH, van der Graaf Y, Grobbee DE, van der Schouw YT. Age at menopause, cause-specific mortality and total life expectancy. Epidemiology. 2005 Jul;**16**(4):556-562

[93] Prolla TA, Mattson MP. Molecular mechanisms of brain aging and neurodegenerative disorders: Lessons from dietary restriction. Trends in Neurosciences. 2001 Nov;**24**(11 Suppl):S21–S31. Review

[94] Ghosh S, Wanders D, Stone KP, Van NT, Cortez CC, Gettys TW. A systems biology analysis of the unique and overlapping transcriptional responses to caloric restriction and dietary methionine restriction in rats. The FASEB Journal. 2014 Jun;**28**(6):2577-2590. DOI: 10.1096/fj.14-249458

[95] Houthoofd K, Braeckman BP, Lenaerts I, Brys K, De Vreese A, Van Eygen S, Vanfleteren JR. No reduction of metabolic rate in food restricted Caenorhabditis elegans. Experimental Gerontology. 2002 Dec;**37**(12):1359-1369

[96] Passarino G, De Rango F, Montesanto A. Human longevity: Genetics or lifestyle? It takes two to tango. Immun Ageing. 2016 Apr 5;**13**:12. DOI: 10.1186/s12979-016-0066-z

[97] Longo VD, Antebi A, Bartke A, Barzilai N, Brown-Borg HM, Caruso C, Curiel TJ, de Cabo R, Franceschi C, Gems D, Ingram DK, Johnson TE, Kennedy BK, Kenyon C, Klein S, Kopchick JJ, Lepperdinger G, Madeo F, Mirisola MG, Mitchell JR, Passarino G, Rudolph KL, Sedivy JM, Shadel GS, Sinclair DA, Spindler SR, Suh Y, Vijg J, Vinciguerra M, Fontana L. Interventions to slow aging in humans: Are we ready?. Aging Cell. 2015 Aug;**14**(4):497-510. DOI: 10.1111/acel.12338. Review

[98] Pes GM, Tolu F, Dore MP, Sechi GP, Errigo A, Canelada A, Poulain M. Male longevity in Sardinia, a review of historical sources supporting a causal link with dietary factors. European Journal of Clinical Nutrition. 2015 Apr;**69**(4):411-418. DOI: 10.1038/ejcn.2014.230. Review

[99] Riccioni G, Bucciarelli T, Mancini B, Di Ilio C, Capra V, D'Orazio N. The role of the antioxidant vitamin supplementation in the prevention of cardiovascular diseases. Expert Opinion on Investigational Drugs. 2007 Jan;**16**(1):25-32

[100] Suzuki M, Willcox DC, Rosenbaum MW, Willcox BJ. Oxidative stress and longevity in okinawa: An investigation of blood lipid peroxidation and tocopherol in okinawan centenarians. Current Gerontology Geriatrics Research. 2010;**2010**:380460. DOI: 10.1155/2010/380460

[101] Paolisso G, Tagliamonte MR, Rizzo MR, Manzella D, Gambardella A, Varricchio M. Oxidative stress and advancing age: Results in healthy centenarians. Journal of the American Geriatrics Society. 1998 Jul;**46**(7):833-838

[102] Willcox DC, Willcox BJ, Todoriki H, Suzuki M. The Okinawan diet: Health implications of a low-calorie, nutrient-dense, antioxidant-rich dietary pattern low in glycemic load. Journal of the American College of Nutrition. 2009 Aug;**28**(Suppl):500S–516S

[103] Arroll B, Beaglehole R. Does physical activity lower blood pressure: A critical review of the clinical trials. Journal of Clinical Epidemiology. 1992 May;**45**(5):439-447

[104] Thompson PD. Exercise and physical activity in the prevention and treatment of atherosclerotic cardiovascular disease. Arteriosclerosis, Thrombosis, and Vascular Biology. 2003 Aug 1;**23**(8):1319-1321

[105] Fulle S, Protasi F, Di Tano G, Pietrangelo T, Beltramin A, Boncompagni S, Vecchiet L, Fanò G. The contribution of reactive oxygen species to sarcopenia and muscle ageing. Experimental Gerontology. 2004 Jan;**39**(1):17-24

[106] Emba RD, Blaum C, Guralnik JM, Moncrief DT, Ricks MO, Fried LP. Carotenoid and vitamin E status are associated with indicators of sarcopenia among older women living in the community. Aging Clinical and Experimental Research. 2003 Dec;**15**(6):482-487

[107] Hu FB, Willett WC, Li T, Stampfer MJ, Colditz GA, Manson JE. Adiposity as compared with physical activity in predicting mortality among women. The New England Journal of Medicine. 2004 Dec 23;**351**(26):2694-2703

[108] Bell JT, Tsai PC, Yang TP, Pidsley R, Nisbet J, Glass D, Mangino M, Zhai G, Zhang F, Valdes A, Shin SY, Dempster EL, Murray RM, Grundberg E, Hedman AK, Nica

A, Small KS; MuTHER Consortium., Dermitzakis ET, McCarthy MI, Mill J, Spector TD, Deloukas P. Epigenome-wide scans identify differentially methylated regions for age and age-related phenotypes in a healthy ageing population. PLoS Genetics. 2012; **8**(4):e1002629. DOI: 10.1371/journal.pgen.1002629

[109] Hernandez DG, Nalls MA, Gibbs JR, Arepalli S, van der Brug M, Chong S, Moore M, Longo DL, Cookson MR, Traynor BJ, Singleton AB. Distinct DNA methylation changes highly correlated with chronological age in the human brain. Human Molecular Genetics. 2011 Mar 15;**20**(6):1164-1172. DOI: 10.1093/hmg/ddq561

[110] Garagnani P, Bacalini MG, Pirazzini C, Gori D, Giuliani C, Mari D, Di Blasio AM, Gentilini D, Vitale G, Collino S, Rezzi S, Castellani G, Capri M, Salvioli S,Franceschi C. Methylation of ELOVL2 gene as a new epigenetic marker of age. Aging Cell. 2012 Dec;**11**(6):1132-1134. DOI: 10.1111/acel.12005

[111] Horvath S. DNA methylation age of human tissues and cell types. Genome Biology. 2013;**14**(10):R115. Erratum in: Genome Biology. 2015;16:96. DOI: 10.1186/gb-2013-14-10-r115

[112] Marioni RE, Shah S, McRae AF, Chen BH, Colicino E, Harris SE, Gibson J, Henders AK, Redmond P, Cox SR, Pattie A, Corley J, Murphy L, Martin NG, Montgomery GW, Feinberg AP, Fallin MD, Multhaup ML, Jaffe AE, Joehanes R, Schwartz J, Just AC, Lunetta KL, Murabito JM, Starr JM, Horvath S, Baccarelli AA, Levy D, Visscher PM, Wray NR, Deary IJ. DNA methylation age of blood predicts all-cause mortality in later life. Genome Biology. 2015 Jan 30;**16**:25. DOI: 10.1186/s13059-015-0584-6

[113] Horvath S, Mah V, Lu AT, Woo JS, Choi OW, Jasinska AJ, Riancho JA, Tung S, Coles NS, Braun J, Vinters HV, Coles LS. The cerebellum ages slowly according to the epigenetic clock. Aging (Albany NY). 2015 May;**7**(5):294-306

[114] Bellizzi D, D'Aquila P, Montesanto A, Corsonello A, Mari V, Mazzei B, Lattanzio F, Passarino G. Global DNA methylation in old subjects is correlated with frailty. Age (Dordrecht, Netherlands). 2012 Feb;**34**(1):169-179. DOI: 10.1007/s11357-011-9216-6

[115] Zhang H, Yang H, Zhang C, Jing Y, Wang C, Liu C, Zhang R, Wang J, Zhang J, Zen K, Zhang C, Li D. Investigation of microRNA expression in human serum during the aging process. J Gerontology A Biological Sciences and Medical Science. 2015 Jan;**70**(1):102-109

[116] Olivieri F, Rippo MR, Prattichizzo F, Babini L, Graciotti L, Recchioni R, Procopio AD. Toll like receptor signaling in "inflammaging": MicroRNA as new players. Immunity & Ageing. 2013 Mar 19;**10**(1):11

[117] Quinn SR, O'Neill LA. A trio of microRNAs that control Toll-like receptor signalling. International Immunology. 2011 Jul;**23**(7):421-425

Chapter 3

Sunflower Leaf Senescence: A Complex Genetic Process with Economic Impact on Crop Production

Sebastián Moschen, Agustín I. López Gialdi,
Norma Paniego, Paula Fernandez and
Ruth Amelia Heinz

Additional information is available at the end of the chapter

http://dx.doi.org/10.5772/intechopen.68588

Abstract

Leaf senescence is a complex process controlled by multiple genetic and environmental variables. In different crops, a delay in leaf senescence has an important impact on grain yield trough the maintenance of the photosynthetic leaf area during the reproductive stage. In sunflower (*Helianthus annuus* L.), the fourth largest oil crop worldwide, senescence reduces the capacity of plants to maintain their green leaf area for longer periods, especially during the grain filling phase, leading to important economic losses.

In crop species, taking into account the temporal gap between the onset and the phenotypic detection of senescence, identification of both, candidate genes and functional stay-green are indispensable to enable the early detection of senescence, the elucidation of molecular mechanisms and the development of tools for breeding applications.

In this chapter a comprehensive literature revision of leaf senescence process not only in model plant species but also in agronomical relevant crops is presented. Results derived from system biology approaches integrating transcriptomic, metabolomic and physiological data as well as those leading to the selection and characterization of stay green sunflower genotypes are included, making an important contribution to the knowledge of leaf senescence process and providing a valuable tool to assist in crop breeding.

Keywords: sunflower, candidate genes, leaf senescence, stay-green genotype, molecular markers

1. Introduction

Leaf senescence is an age-dependent complex process at the cellular, tissue, organ or organism level, leading to death at the end of the life span [1]. Annual plants as grain and oil crops undergo a visual process toward the end of the reproductive stage that is accompanied by nutrient remobilization from leaf to developing seeds [2]. Senescence process is controlled by multiple genetic and environmental variables, which has strong impact on crop yield [3]. Environmental factors such as light, nutrient availability, concentration of CO_2, abiotic and biotic stresses caused by disease may affect the rate of senescence. In this context, not only environmental conditions but also biotic factors influence senescence, being this an irreversible process prematurely induced under these adverse conditions [4]. Moreover, reproductive growth is mentioned as a factor that usually impacts on leaf senescence, and particularly in sunflower, the lack of sinks delays the onset of senescence [5]. During this process, changes in gene expression result in a metabolic shift from anabolism to catabolism, which leads to decreased photosynthetic activity, progressive degradation of cellular structures and oxidative burst [6–8]. It has been documented that a delay in leaf senescence has a substantial impact on grain yield through the maintenance of the photosynthetic leaf area during the reproductive stage in different crops [3, 9, 10].

In sunflower (*Helianthus annuus* L.), the largest important oil crop worldwide, the senescence process reduces the capacity of plants to maintain their green leaf area for longer periods, especially during the grain-filling phase, affecting the yield and thus leading to economic losses [11, 12]. This production constraint has deepened since sunflower crop production has been gradually moved to marginal areas due to the rapid change of agricultural practices in crops such as soybean and maize, which have greatly increased their cultivated areas as a consequence of favorable commodity prices and because farmers found more profitable to sow transgenic crops with resistance to herbicides and insects [13, 14].

During the last years, many efforts have been achieved to build up useful functional genomics tools for cultivated sunflower involving physiological, transcriptional and metabolic profiles [15–23].

In crop species, considering the temporal gap between onset and phenotypic detection of senescence process, the availability of candidate genes and molecular markers to the early detection of senescence is indispensable to discriminate between early-senescing and late-senescing lines to be applied in the different context of breeding activities [24]. For example, the identification of functional stay-green genotypes for breeding applications and/or for elucidating molecular mechanisms involved in this complex trait.

2. Senescence and crop yields: stay-green genotypes

Senescence is an essential process for the normal growth and development of plants, being an important mechanism for the adaptation to several environmental conditions.

The hypothesis that a delay leaf senescence increases the productivity may be valid for most crops with regard to total biomass production and tuber crops, but this assumption is more controversial with respect to seed yields [3]. However, it has been documented that a delay in leaf senescence has a high impact on grain weight and quality in different crops, including sunflower [3, 5, 25, 26].

Stay-green is a regular term given to genotypes in which the senescence phenotype is delayed in comparison with a standard reference genotype. Stay-green genotypes could be classified into five different types taking into consideration functional or cosmetic stay-green [27, 28]. Functional stay-green genotypes have a photosynthetically active leaf area showing a delay in the onset of senescence (class A), or differing in the rate of the process (class B), whereas cosmetic stay-green genotypes are those in which the senescence proceeds normally but they show problems in chlorophyll degradation (class C), or the chlorophyll content does not decline due to rapid tissue death (class D), or they have a higher chlorophyll content with no change in onset or rate of senescence development (class E) [28]. Mature leaf is a net contributor of photosynthates to the whole plant. The carbon capture phase of the leaf is followed by a net organic nitrogen remobilization. The transition from carbon capture to nitrogen remobilization corresponds to the functional initiation of senescence [29]. In this sense, functional stay-green genotypes are present in those genotypes in which the C–N transition is delayed, or the transition occurs but the subsequent yellowing and N remobilization run slowly [29–31].

In this sense, functional stay-green genotypes could intercept more radiation, increasing photosynthesis and yield in crops with seeds rich in carbon compounds. However, a delay in the C–N transition could negatively affect the seed quality in crops with seed rich in protein compounds [30], such as soybean [32] and cowpea [33].

3. Study of leaf senescence process in sunflower

Sunflower is the fourth most important oil crop worldwide and the second one in the Argentine. Moreover, Argentina is the third largest exporter of crude oil and the second of protein and pellet flour. The added value of oilseed industrialization contributes in the economy with US$ 1400 million approximately, with a total production between 3.2 and 3.8 million tons of grain annually [34].

Sunflower is an annual monocarpic species in which reproductive phase exerts a strong control on leaf senescence and nutrient remobilization, affecting grain weight [35]. Potential yields of sunflower crop are far from the real ones in all Argentina productive regions. In Balcarce location, for instance (Southeast of Buenos Aires province), one of the best productive regions of Argentina, while the potential yields are estimated in 5000 kg ha^{-1}, those obtained by the best producers only reach 3000 kg ha^{-1}, and the average in the region ranges in 1800 kg ha^{-1} [36]. Among the factors that contribute to the productivity gap, one of the most important is the inability of current hybrids to keep their green leaf area for long periods, limiting the incident radiation capture during the grain-filling period and impacting negatively on the yield and oil concentration [12, 37].

Sunflower genome complexity characterized by of long and highly similar repeats has slowed the pace of getting a complete genome reference. Recently, a high-quality assembly comprising 3.6 Gigabases has being achieved by means of PACBIO sequencing [38]. The reference genome together with extensive transcriptomic data from vegetative and floral organs is accessible at https://www.heliagene.org/HanXRQ-SUNRISE. In the last years, our group accomplished a series of transcriptional and metabolic profiling studies that were integrated into physiological, molecular and cytological analysis to contribute to the understanding the senescence process in this crop and breeding genotypes against abiotic constraints [19–23, 39–41].

Through a system biology approach and using a commercial sunflower hybrid, we characterized the leaf senescence process by integrating transcriptomic and metabolomic analyses using both glasshouse and field conditions [22]. Our results revealed early metabolic changes before to anthesis in the absence of the onset of the first visual senescence symptoms, with more pronounced changes observed when physiological and molecular variables were assessed under field conditions (**Figure 1**). Metabolite remobilization from mature and senescent leaves to the different sinks, particularly into seed development, affects their quality and quantity and is one of the most important aspects of crop improvement [3]. In this study, we showed a decrease of photosynthetic activity and cell growth before anthesis, whereas sucrose, fatty acid, nucleotide and amino acid metabolisms increased. The role of sugars in senescence has been widely discussed in recent years. Sugars are central elements of the source-sink relationships [42, 43] and have been reported as growth [44] and photosynthetic rate regulators [45]. However, the effect of sugars on senescence is controversial and differs between different species [1, 46, 47]. In sunflower, sugar content decreases during leaf development (**Figure 1**). This finding is in line with previous studies in tomato and higher plants, in which the photosynthetic rate dropped together with sugar levels in a mature leaf [48–50]. Furthermore, sunflower is a plant with a high demand for nutrient, especially sugars as substrate for oil synthesis, during the grain-filling phase. Likewise, low levels of sugars may increase production and/or ethylene sensitivity, which acts as senescence enhancer [51, 52].

Pathways related to nutrient recycling processes were also up-regulated. We found high expression levels of enzymes involved in recycling, such as asparagine synthetase and glutamine synthase, as well as the associated metabolites, asparagine and glutamine. These amino acids are involved in nitrogen and carbon transport between the different organs and are the most abundant amino acids in the xylem and phloem [53, 54], indicating a high recycling activity at early stages of leaf development.

Transcription factors (TFs) are key proteins involved in the regulation of gene expression and signal transduction networks, regulating different biological processes and their function is crucial for triggering and/or controlling the different aspect of senescence process. Members of the NAC, AP2-EREBP, HB, bZIP and MYB transcription factor families showed high expression levels, and their expression level was highly correlated, suggesting their involvement in sunflower senescence. These results are in agreement with previous results described for *Arabidopsis thaliana* [55]. Particularly, we found a transcript with high sequence identity

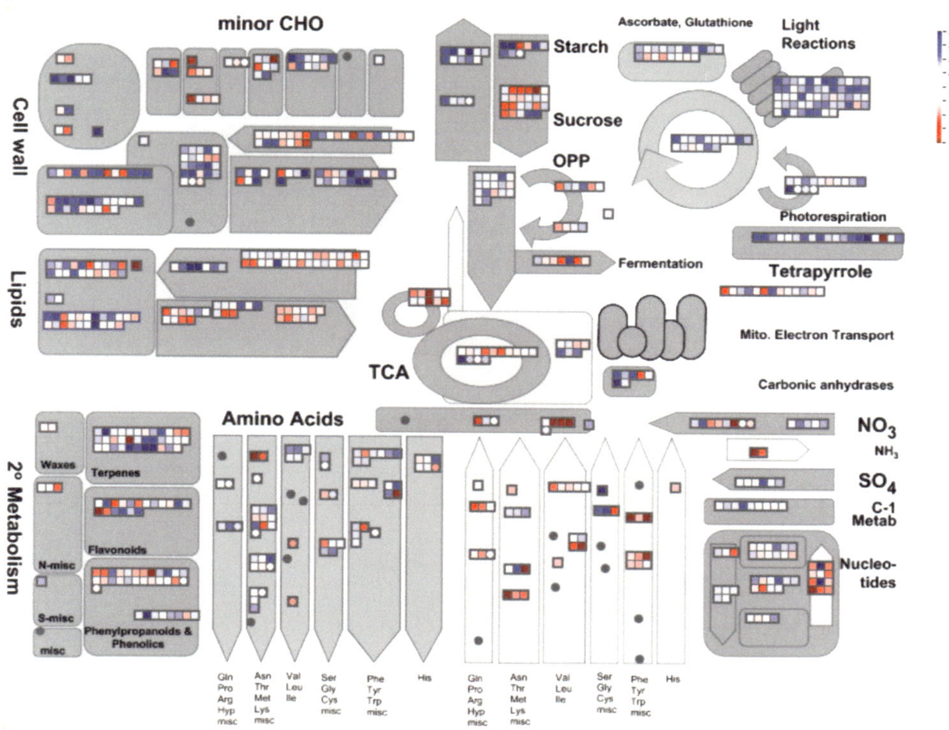

Figure 1. Metabolism overview in the field experiment at pre-anthesis time. Genes and metabolites are represented by squares and circles, respectively. Color intensity corresponds to the expression ratio at logarithmic scale (red: up-regulated, blue: down-regulated) [22].

to *ANAC02* or *ATAF1*. This transcript might be associated with an upstream regulation of the signaling pathway involving ORE1 and EIN2 [56], thus activating their expression and inhibiting the expression of Golden2-like (GLKs) genes, which are necessary for chloroplast development and maintenance [57]. ORE1 also acts as an antagonist of GLK protein, adding more complexity to this regulation pathway [57]. In *A. thaliana*, ORE1 TF induces leaf senescence [58]. In addition, the micro-RNA *miR164* suppress *ORE1* transcript levels; *miR164* and *ORE1* may be regulated in a loop that would also involve EIN2, where EIN2 would promote the expression of ORE1 and would inhibit *miR164* [59]. In a previous work conducted in sunflower, expression profiles of candidate genes *Ha-EIN2* and *Ha-NAC01* (with high sequence identity to *ORE1*) were evaluated together with *miR164* levels [21] showing similar expression patterns to Arabidopsis and in line with the increase in the nutrient remobilization rate.

Moreover, using bioinformatic approaches and evaluating two different approaches for gene expression correlation analysis: Weighted Gene Correlation Network Analysis (WGCNA) and BioSignature Discoverer (BioSD, Gnosis Data Analysis, Heraklion, Greece), we integrated transcriptomic and metabolomic data [39]. WGCNA allowed the detection of 10 metabolites and 13 TFs (**Figure 2**), whereas BioSD allowed the detection of one metabolite and six TFs as potential biomarkers. Comparative analysis demonstrated that three transcription factors were detected

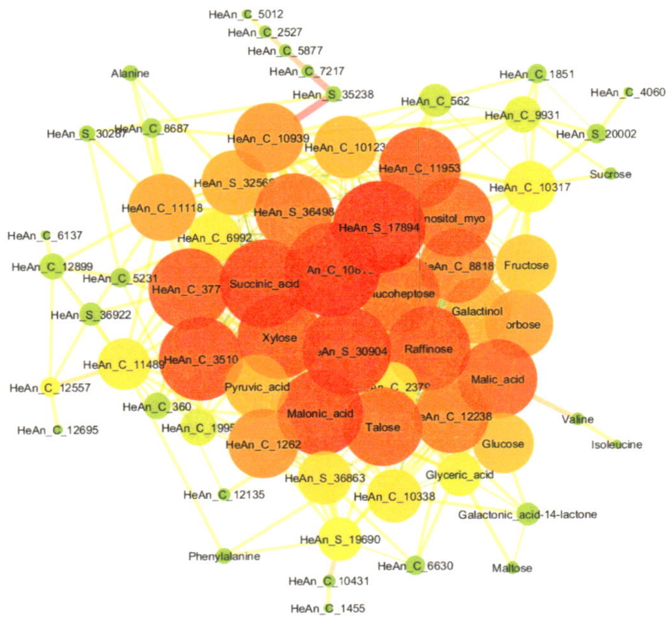

Figure 2. Integrated network of hubs metabolites and transcription factors detected by WGCNA [39]. 24 selected hubs metabolites and 82 TFs statistically significant during senescence were correlated (p-value < 0.0001) and visualized in Cytoscape [60] by degree (node size and color) and edge weight (edge size and color).

by both approaches, highlighting them as potentially robust biomarkers associated with leaf senescence in sunflower. This complementary use of network and BioSignature Discoverer analysis of transcriptomic and metabolomic data provided a useful tool for identifying candidate genes and metabolites, which may have a role in the triggering and development of the leaf senescence process.

Transcriptomic analysis in combination with metabolic profile is a comprenhensive tool for the study of leaf senescence. These results suggest a complex regulatory network underlying this process. Thus, the identification of regulatory networks based on expression profiling is an important starting point for the detection of new key genes involved in the triggering of the senescence process in this crop.

4. Selection of stay-green genotypes in sunflower

Given the importance of the stay-green genotypes selection for studies of this complex character, we performed a screening and selection of contrasting sunflower genotypes associated with early leaf senescence process evaluating 135 different genotypes from the INTA Sunflower Breeding Program (INTA Manfredi Sunflower Germplasm Collection) [61] growing under field conditions through a physiological, cytological and molecular approach.

Physiological measurement of growing cycle, anthesis time, number of leaves, plant size, evolution of total/dry leaf, green leaf area at anthesis time and SPAD was performed to select pairs of contrasting genotypes with very similar plant architecture, phenology and leaf area until anthesis, but with different senescence rate. This analysis allowed us to select 10 genotypes that were further evaluated, allowing the identification of two contrasting senescence inbred lines, R453 (early senescence genotype) and B481-6 (putative stay-green genotype) [23] (**Figure 3**).

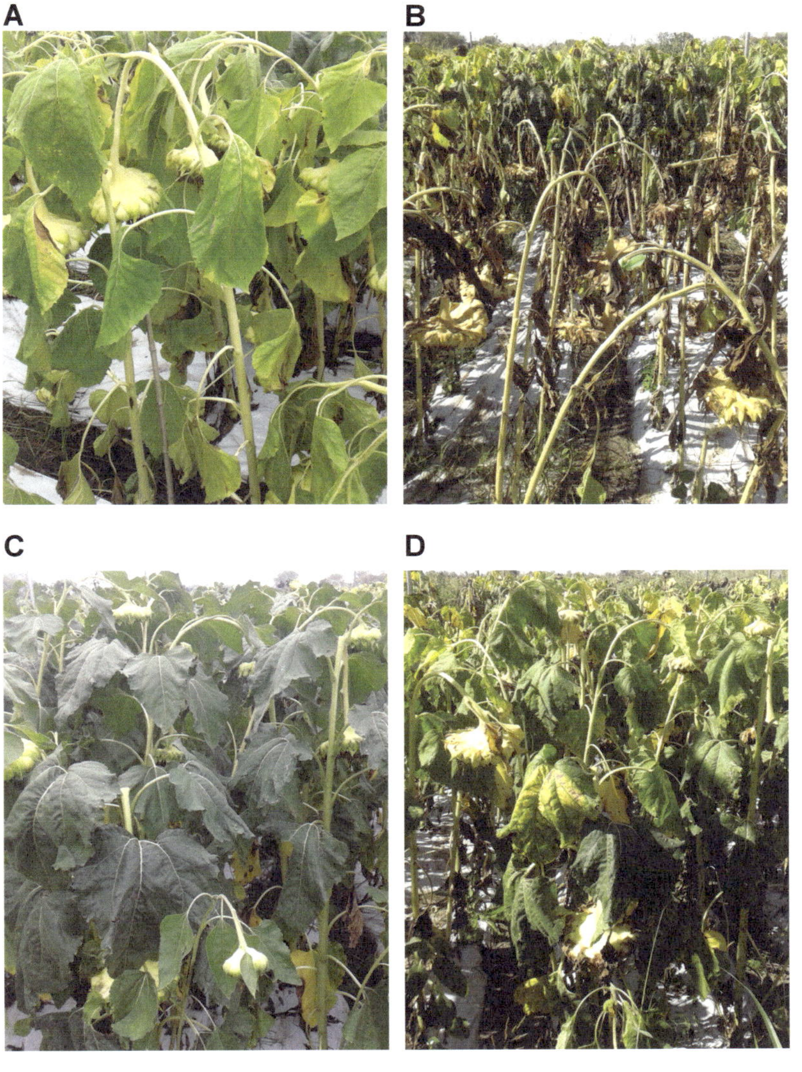

Figure 3. Phenotypic analysis of sunflower genotypes under field experiment. (A) and (B) early senescence genotype R453. (C) and (D) Stay-green genotype B481-6. Images (A) and (C) correspond to 15 days after anthesis and images (B) and (D) 30 days after anthesis.

At the physiological level, green leaf area evolution (GLA) is an indirect measurement of photosynthetically active leaf area, and its decrease has been reported as product of active chloroplast degeneration and chlorophyll degradation.

R453 and B481-6 displayed similar GLA evolution until anthesis. Then, GLA decreased abruptly in R453 and faster than the B481-6 genotype. GLA decline in B481-6, on the other hand, was gradual and reached complete senescence at 200 ºCdAE later (**Figure 4A**). In sunflower, and many other monocarpic species, this senescence symptom is evident after anthesis, during grain-filling period, and is mainly due to source-sink relationships established at this stage of development [5, 20, 36, 62]. Radiation interception at the canopy level showed similar patterns with an early decrease in the early senescence genotype (**Figure 4C**). In grain crops, a delay in leaf senescence should have a positive impact on grain yield [3, 26]. Yield components were evaluated displaying significant differences in yield, with higher seed weight in the stay-green genotype (**Figure 4B**). These observations are in agreement with the expected for this trait suggesting a type B stay-green phenotype [28]. Moreover, photosynthesis measurement was performed 15 days after anthesis showing higher photosynthesis rate in the stay-green genotype (**Figure 4D**), supporting this finding.

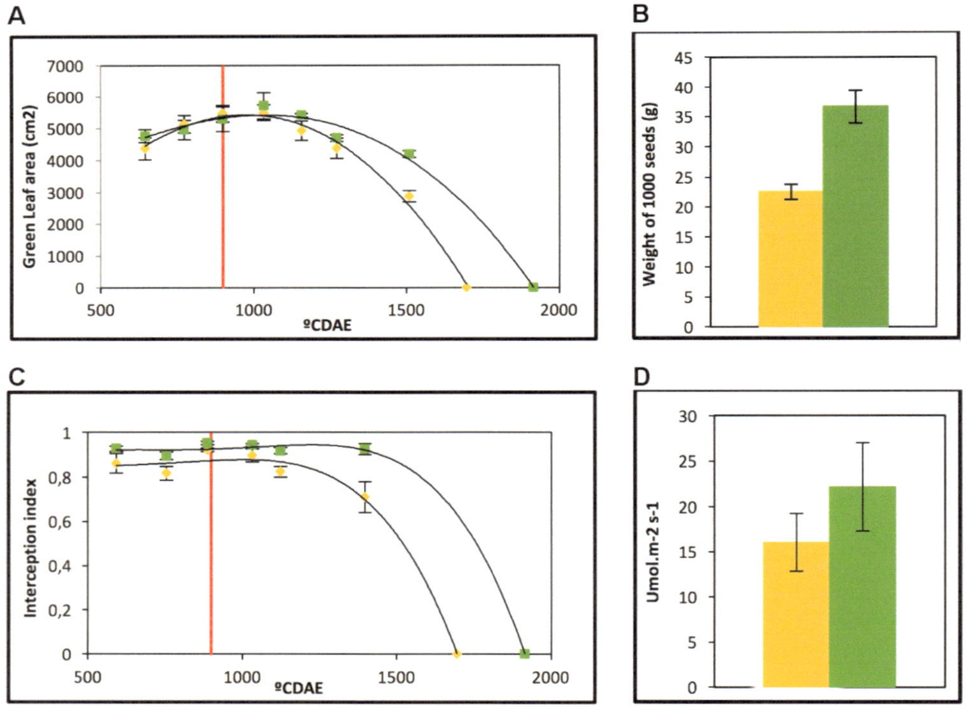

Figure 4. Physiological analysis of contrasting genotypes. R453 in orange and B481-6 in green colors. (A) Green leaf area (GLA); (B) yield; (C) radiation interception and (D) photosynthesis. ºCdAE indicates thermal time after emergence. Red line in (A) and (C) indicates anthesis time for both genotypes.

To confirm the senescence phenotype of the selected genotypes, we also performed cytological and molecular analysis. As senescence involves programed Cell Death (PCD), nuclear DNA degradation associated with PCD can be detected in situ by TUNEL assay. In this sense, we analyzed mesophyll cells nuclei of both genotypes 10 days after anthesis. R453, with premature senescence phenotype, also showed TUNEL-positive nuclei, whereas B481-6, with stay-green phenotype, had TUNEL-negative nuclei (**Figure 5**). Mesophyll is the most photosynthetically active tissue of higher plants, having cells with high chloroplast and chlorophyll content and the cells in this tissue are affected firstly during senescence [9, 62, 63]. TUNEL-positive nuclei detection indicates that senescence process has already started in the early senescence genotype.

The gene expression pattern of the senescence-associated candidate transcription factors was evaluated for differences in the timing of senescence pathways activation between the early senescence and stay-green genotype [21, 22]. HaNAC01, HaNAC03 and HaNAC05 transcription factors were evaluated at two different times, 5 days after anthesis (DAA) and 15 days after anthesis (**Figure 6**). R453 showed higher expression levels of the three NAC transcription factor than B481-6, and its expression increased by 15 days post-anthesis.

Altogether, these findings highlight these genotypes as interesting potential candidates for further analysis of leaf senescence in sunflower. The B481-6 genotype showed a stay-green phenotype, also evidenced by cytological and molecular analysis and an increase of seed weight,

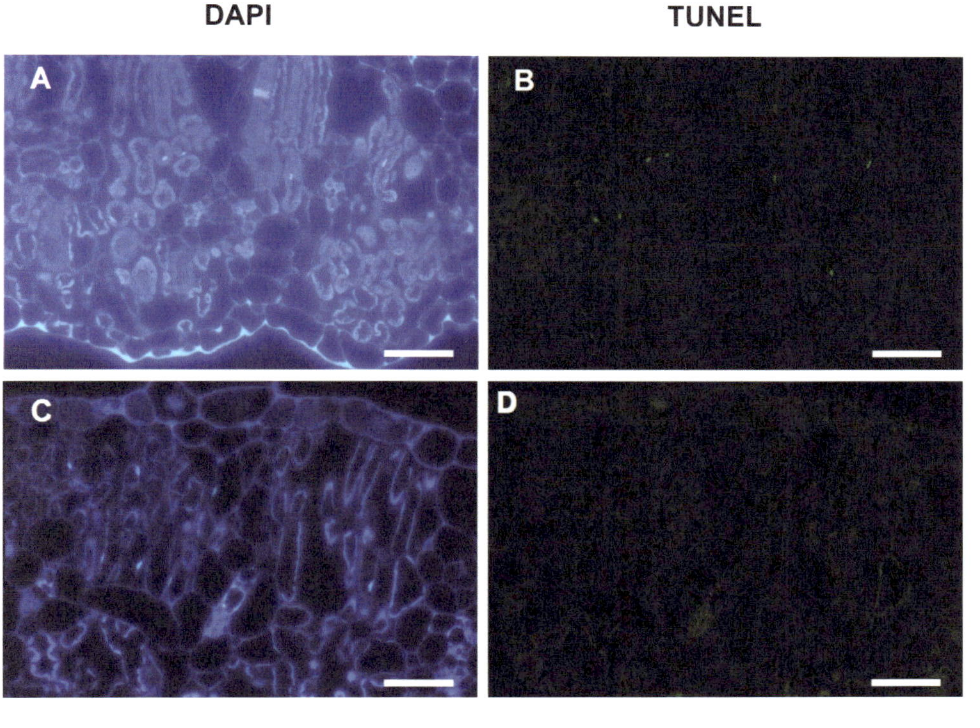

Figure 5. TUNEL assays of selected contrasting genotypes. (A) and (C): Nuclei visualization by DAPI staining. (B): TUNEL-positive nuclei in mesophyll cells of premature senescence genotypes (R453). (D): TUNEL-negative nuclei in stay-green genotype (B481-6) [23].

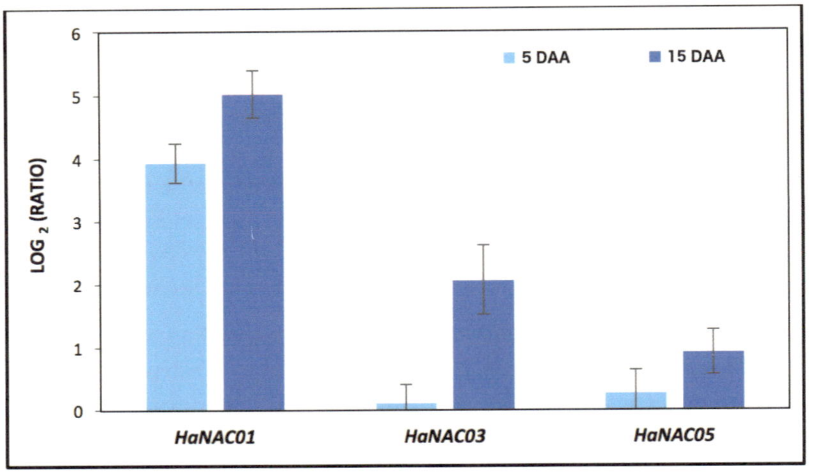

Figure 6. qPCR analysis of NAC transcription factors candidate genes. Relative transcript levels are shown as the ratio (log2 scale) between the expression in the early senescence genotype (R453) in relation to the stay-green genotype (B481-6) in two different times 5 days after anthesis (DAA) and 15 days after anthesis [23].

which makes this genotype a potential candidate for the functional stay-green phenotype in comparison with R453 genotype.

5. Conclusions and perspectives

Integration of transcriptomic and metabolomics data arises as a powerful approach to identify pathways and candidate genes related to the senescence process in sunflower, an economically important oil crop without previous molecular information about this process. The results discussed in this chapter provide an important start point for understanding the senescence process and open new insights to explore alternative strategies and possibilities.

Moreover, by a combination of physiological, cytological and molecular analysis, we identified two senescence contrasting genotypes. B481-6 genotype showed a delay in senescence symptom evaluated both, under physiological and molecular measurement. This senescence delay, together with an increase in photosynthesis rate, leads to an increase in yield, highlighting this genotype as functional stay-green. These results together with a better understanding of the onset of the process will in turn impact on the development of different senescence management strategies and could help controlling the grain-filling process. All in all, these advances provide a valuable tool to assist in crop breeding, which represents a significant challenge for the future of agriculture attending to the increase in both, world population and climate risks that affect productivity.

Acknowledgements

This research was supported by Research Projects of the Instituto Nacional de Tecnología Agropecuaria (INTA), ANPCyT and CONICET (MINCyT) and the DEANN Project (UE). Dr.

S. Moschen holds a postdoctoral fellowship from CONICET, Lic. A. I. López Gialdi holds a doctoral fellowship from CONICET, whereas Dr. N. Paniego, Dr. P. Fernandez, Dr. R. A. Heinz are career members of the Consejo Nacional de Investigaciones Científicas y Técnicas (CONICET, Argentina) and INTA researchers.

Author details

Sebastián Moschen[1,2,3], Agustín I. López Gialdi[2], Norma Paniego[1,2], Paula Fernandez[1,2,3] and Ruth Amelia Heinz[1,2,4]*

*Address all correspondence to: heinz.ruth@inta.gob.ar

1 Instituto de Biotecnología, CICVyA, Instituto Nacional de Tecnología Agropecuaria, Hurlingham, Buenos Aires, Argentina

2 Consejo Nacional de Investigaciones Científicas y Técnicas, CONICET, Ciudad Autónoma de Buenos Aires, Argentina

3 Escuela de Ciencia y Tecnología, Universidad Nacional de San Martín, San Martín, Buenos Aires, Argentina

4 Facultad de Ciencias Exactas y Naturales, Universidad de Buenos Aires, Ciudad Autónoma de Buenos Aires, Argentina

References

[1] Nooden LD. Whole plant senescence. In: AC L, editor. Senescence and Aging in Plants. San Diego, USA: Academic Press; 1988. pp. 392-439

[2] Buchanan-Wollaston V, Earl S, Harrison E, Mathas E, Navabpour S, Page T, et al. The molecular analysis of leaf senescence--a genomics approach. Plant Biotechnology Journal. 2003;**1**:3-22. DOI: 10.1046/j.1467-7652.2003.00004.x

[3] Gregersen PL, Culetic A, Boschian L, Krupinska K. Plant senescence and crop productivity. Plant Molecular Biology. 2013;**82**:603-622. DOI: 10.1007/s11103-013-0013-8

[4] Lim PO, Woo HR, Nam HG. Molecular genetics of leaf senescence in Arabidopsis. Trends in Plant Science. 2003;**8**:272-278. DOI: 10.1016/S1360-1385(03)00103-1

[5] Sadras VO, Echarte L, Andrade FH. Profiles of leaf senescence during reproductive growth of sunflower and maize. Annals of Botany. 2000;**85**:187-195

[6] Guo Y, Cai Z, Gan S. Transcriptome of Arabidopsis leaf senescence. Plant, Cell & Environment. 2004;**27**:521-549

[7] Agüera E, Cabello P, de la Haba P. Induction of leaf senescence by low nitrogen nutrition in sunflower (*Helianthus annuus*) plants. Physiologia Plantarum. 2010;**138**:256-267. DOI: 10.1111/j.1399-3054.2009.01336.x

[8] Srivalli B, Khanna-Chopra R. The developing reproductive "sink" induces oxidative stress to mediate nitrogen mobilization during monocarpic senescence in wheat. Biochemical and Biophysical Research Communications. 2004;**325**:198-202. DOI: 10.1016/j.bbrc.2004.09.221

[9] Thomas H. Senescence, ageing and death of the whole plant. New Phytol. 2013;**197**: 696-711. doi:10.1111/nph.12047

[10] Kusaba M, Tanaka A, Tanaka R. Stay-green plants: What do they tell us about the molecular mechanism of leaf senescence. Photosynthesis Research. 2013;**117**:221-234. DOI: 10.1007/s11120-013-9862-x

[11] Aguirrezabal LAN, Lavaud Y, Dosio GAA, Izquierdo NG, Andrade FH, González LM. Intercepted solar radiation during seedlling determines sunflower weight per seed and oil concentration. Crop Science. 2003;**161**:152-161

[12] Dosio GAA, Aguirrezabal LAN, Andrade FH, Pereyra VR. Solar radiation intercepted during seed filling and oil production in two sunflower hybrids. Crop Science. 2000;**1644**: 1637-1644

[13] Moschen S, Radonic LM, Ehrenbolger GF, Fernández P, Lía V, Paniego NB, et al. Functional genomics and transgenesis applied to sunflower breeding. In: Arribas JI, editor. Sunflowers: Growth and Development, Environmental Influences and Pests/Diseases. Nova Science Publishers Inc., New York; 2014. pp. 131-164

[14] Debaeke P, Casadebaig P, Flenet F, Langlade N. Sunflower crop and climate change: Vulnerability, adaptation, and mitigation potential from case-studies in Europe. OCL. EDP Sciences. 2017; **24**:1-15. DOI: 10.1051/ocl/2016052

[15] Fernandez P, Paniego N, Lew S, Hopp HE, Heinz RA. Differential representation of sunflower ESTs in enriched organ-specific cDNA libraries in a small scale sequencing project. BMC Genomics. 2003;**4**:40. DOI: 10.1186/1471-2164-4-40

[16] Paniego N, Heinz RA, Fernandez P, Talia P, Nishinakamasu V, Hopp HE. Sunflower. In: Kole C, editor. Genome Mapping and Molecular Breeding in Plants. Berlin Heidelberg: Springer-Verlag; 2007. pp. 153-177. DOI: 10.1007/978-3-540-34388-2_4

[17] Fernandez P, Rienzo J Di, Fernandez L, Hopp HE, Paniego N, Heinz RA, et al. Transcriptomic identification of candidate genes involved in sunflower responses to chilling and salt stresses based on cDNA microarray analysis. BMC Plant Biology. 2008;**8**:1-18. DOI: 10.1186/1471-2229-8-11

[18] Peluffo L, Lia V, Troglia C, Maringolo C, Norma P, Escande A, et al. Metabolic profiles of sunflower genotypes with contrasting response to *Sclerotinia sclerotiorum* infection. Phytochemistry. Elsevier Ltd. 2010;**71**:70-80. DOI: 10.1016/j.phytochem.2009.09.018

[19] Fernandez P, Soria M, Blesa D, DiRienzo J, Moschen S, Rivarola M, et al. Development, characterization and experimental validation of a cultivated sunflower (*Helianthus annuus* L.) gene expression oligonucleotide microarray. PLoS One. 2012;**7**:1-11. DOI: 10.1371/journal.pone.0045899

[20] Fernandez P, Moschen S, Paniego N, Heinz RA. Functional approaches to study leaf senescence in sunflower. In: Nagata T, editor. Senescence. InTech Open Access Publisher, Croatia; 2012. pp. 69-88. DOI: 10.5772/1905

[21] Moschen S, Bengoa Luoni S, Paniego NB, Hopp HE, Dosio GAA, Fernandez P, et al. Identication of candidate genes associated with leaf senescence in cultivated sunflower (Helianthus annuus L.). PLoS One. 2014;9:e104379. DOI: 10.1371/journal.pone.0104379

[22] Moschen S, Bengoa Luoni S, Di Rienzo J, Caro M, Tohge T, Watanabe M, et al. Integrating transcriptomic and metabolomic analysis to understand natural leaf senescence in sunflower. Plant Biotechnology Journal. 2016;**14**:719-734. DOI: 10.1111/pbi.12422

[23] López Gialdi AI, Moschen S, Villán CS, López Fernández MP, Maldonado S, Paniego N, et al. Identification and characterization of contrasting sunflower genotypes to early leaf senescence process combining molecular and physiological studies (*Helianthus annuus* L.). Plant Sciences. 2016;**250**:40-50. DOI: 10.1016/j.plantsci.2016.05.017

[24] Diaz C, Purdy S, Christ A, Morot-Gaudry J-F, Wingler A, Masclaux-Daubresse C. Characterization of Markers to Determine the Extent and Variability of Leaf Senescence in Arabidopsis. A Metabolic Profiling Approach 1. Plant Physiology. 2005;**138**:898-908. DOI: 10.1104/pp.105.060764.898

[25] De la Vega AJ, Cantore Ma., Sposaro MM, Trápani N, López Pereira M, Hall AJ. Canopy stay-green and yield in non-stressed sunflower. Field Crops Research. 2011;**121**:175-185. DOI: 10.1016/j.fcr.2010.12.015

[26] Gregersen PL. Senescence and nutrient remobilization in crop plants. In: Hawkesford MJ, Barraclough P, editors. The Molecular and Physiological Basis of Nutrient Use Efficiency in Crops. Oxford, UK: Wiley-Blackwell; 2011. pp. 83-102

[27] Thomas H, Smart CM. Crops that stay green. Annals of Applied Biology. Blackwell Publishing Ltd. 1993;**123**:193-219. DOI: 10.1111/j.1744-7348.1993.tb04086.x

[28] Thomas H, Howarth CJ. Five ways to stay green. Journal of Experimental Botany. 2000;**51**:329-337

[29] Thomas H, Ougham H. Senescence and crop performance. In: Sadras V, Calderini D, editors. Applications for Genetic Improvement, Agronomy and Farming Systems. 2nd ed. New York: Crop Physiology; 2014

[30] Thomas H, Ougham H. The stay-green trait. Journal of Experimental Botany. 2014;**65**: 3889-3900. DOI: 10.1093/jxb/eru037

[31] Yoo S-C, Cho S-H, Zhang H, Paik H-C, Lee C-H, Li J, et al. Quantitative trait loci associated with functional stay-green SNU-SG1 in rice. Molecules and Cells. 2007;**24**:83-94. Available: http://www.ncbi.nlm.nih.gov/pubmed/17846502

[32] Kumudini S. Trials and tribulations: A review of the role of assimilate supply in soybean genetic yield improvement. Field Crops Research. 2002;**75**:211-222. DOI: 10.1016/S0378-4290(02)00027-8

[33] Ismail AM, Hall AE, Ehlers JD. Delayed-Leaf-Senescence and Heat-Tolerance Traits Mainly Are Independently Expressed in Cowpea. Crop Science. 2000;**40**:1049-1055.

[34] ASAGIR. Asociación Argentina de Girasol [Internet]. Available: www.asagir.org.ar

[35] López Pereira M, Sadras VO, Trápani N. Genetic improvement of sunflower in Argentina between 1930 and 1995. I. Yield and its Components. Field Crops Research. 1999;**62**:157-166.

[36] Dosio GAA, Aguirrezábal LAN. Variaciones del rendimiento en girasol. Identificando las causas. Revista Agromercado, Cuadernillo de girasol. 2004;**90**:7-10

[37] Aguirrezábal LAN, Lavaud Y, Dosio GAA, Izquierdo NG, Andrade FH, González LM. Weight per seed and oil concentration in a sunflower hybrid are accounted for by intercepted solar radiation during a definite period of seed filling. Crop Science. 2003;**43**:152-161

[38] Gouzy J, Mayjonade B, Grassa C, Carrere S, Sallet E, Legrand L, et al. Result of the de novo Sequencing of the Complex Sunflower Genome Using PacBio Technology (100X). XXIV Plant & Animal Genome Conference; San Diego, CA; 2016

[39] Moschen S, Higgins J, Di Rienzo JA, Heinz RA, Paniego N, Fernandez P, et al. Network and biosignature analysis for the integration of transcriptomic and metabolomic data to characterize leaf senescence process in sunflower. BMC Bioinformatics. BioMed Central. 2016;**17**:174. DOI: 10.1186/s12859-016-1045-2

[40] de la Mata L, Cabello P, de la Haba P, Agüera E. Growth under elevated atmospheric CO2 concentration accelerates leaf senescence in sunflower (*Helianthus annuus* L.) plants. Journal of Plant Physiology. 2012;**169**:1392-1400

[41] Agüera E, Cabello P, de la Mata L, Molina E, de la Haba P. Metabolic Regulation of Leaf Senescence in Sunflower (*Helianthus annuus* L.) Plants. In: Nagata T, editor. Senescence. InTech Open Access Publisher, Croatia; 2012. pp. 51-68. DOI: 10.5772/1905.

[42] Balibrea Lara ME, Gonzalez Garcia M-C, Fatima T, Ehness R, Lee TK, Proels R, et al. Extracellular invertase is an essential component of cytokinin-mediated delay of senescence. The Plant Cell. 2004;**16**:1276-1287. DOI: 10.1105/tpc.018929

[43] Roitsch T, González M-C. Function and regulation of plant invertases: Sweet sensations. Trends in Plant Science. 2004;**9**:606-613. DOI: 10.1016/j.tplants.2004.10.009

[44] Smeekens S, Ma J, Hanson J, Rolland F. Sugar signals and molecular networks controlling plant growth. Current Opinion in Plant Biology. Elsevier Ltd. 2010;**13**:274-279. DOI: 10.1016/j.pbi.2009.12.002

[45] Wingler A, Von Schaewen A, Leegood RC, Lea PL, Quick PW. Regulation of leaf senescence by cytokinin, sugars, and light. Plant Physiology. 1998;**116**:329-335

[46] Wingler A, Masclaux-Daubresse C, Fischer AM. Sugars, senescence, and ageing in plants and heterotrophic organisms. Journal of Experimental Botany. 2009;**60**:1063-1066. DOI: 10.1093/jxb/erp067

[47] Yoshida S. Molecular regulation of leaf senescence. Current Opinion in Plant Biology. 2003;**6**:79-84. DOI: 10.1016/S1369-5266(02)00009-2

[48] Quirino BF, Noh YS, Himelblau E, Amasino RM. Molecular aspects of leaf senescence. Trends in Plant Science. 2000;**5**:278-282. Available: http://www.ncbi.nlm.nih.gov/pubmed/10871899

[49] Jang JC, León P, Zhou L, Sheen J. Hexokinase as a sugar sensor in higher plants. Plant Cell Online. 1997;**9**:5-19. DOI: 10.1105/tpc.9.1.5

[50] Dai N, Schaffer A, Petreikov M, Shahak Y, Giller Y, Ratner K, et al. Overexpression of Arabidopsis hexokinase in tomato plants inhibits growth, reduces photosynthesis, and induces rapid senescence. The Plant Cell. 1999;**11**:1253-1266. Available: http://www.ncbi.nlm.nih.gov/pubmed/10402427

[51] Grbic V, Bleecker AB. Ethylene regulates the timing of leaf senescence in Arabidopsis. The Plant Journal. 1995;**8**:595-602. DOI: 10.1046/j.1365-313X.1995.8040595.x

[52] Hoeberichts FA, van Doorn WG, Vorst O, Hall RD, van Wordragen MF. Sucrose prevents up-regulation of senescence-associated genes in carnation petals. Journal of Experimental Botany. 2007;**58**:2873-2885. DOI: 10.1093/jxb/erm076

[53] Lea P, Miflin B. Transport and Metabolism of Asparagine and Other Nitrogen Compounds within the Plant. In: Miflin B, editor. The Biochemistry of Plants. Vol. 5. Amino Acids and Derivatives. Academic Press, New York, 569-607.

[54] Urquhart AA, Joy KW. Use of Phloem exudate technique in the study of amino Acid transport in pea plants. Plant Physiology. 1981;**68**:750-754. Available: http://www.pubmedcentral.nih.gov/articlerender.fcgi?artid=425975&tool=pmcentrez&rendertype=abstract

[55] Balazadeh S, Riaño-Pachón DM, Mueller-Roeber B. Transcription factors regulating leaf senescence in *Arabidopsis thaliana*. Plant Biology. 2008;**10**:63-75. DOI: 10.1111/j.1438-8677.2008.00088.x

[56] Balazadeh S, Garapati P, Xue G, Mueller-Roeber B. A transcription factor upstream of ORE1 and GLK1 integrates ABA signalling with drought-induced senescence. 6th European Workshop on Leaf Senescence 14-18 October INRA, Versailles, France. 2013

[57] Rauf M, Arif M, Dortay H, Matallana-Ramírez LP, Waters MT, Gil Nam H, et al. ORE1 balances leaf senescence against maintenance by antagonizing G2-like-mediated transcription. EMBO Reports. 2013;**14**:382-388. DOI: 10.1038/embor.2013.24

[58] Balazadeh S, Siddiqui H, Allu AD, Matallana-Ramirez LP, Caldana C, Mehrnia M, et al. A gene regulatory network controlled by the NAC transcription factor ANAC092/AtNAC2/ORE1 during salt-promoted senescence. Plant Journal. 2010;**62**:250-264. DOI: TPJ4151 [pii] 10.1111/j.1365-313X.2010.04151.x

[59] Kim JH, Woo HR, Kim J, Lim PO, Lee IC, Choi SH, et al. Trifurcate feed-forward regulation of age-dependent cell death involving miR164 in Arabidopsis. Science. 2009;**323**:1053-1057. DOI: 10.1126/science.1166386

[60] Shannon P, Markiel A, Ozier O, Baliga NS, Wang JT, Ramage D, et al. Cytoscape: A software environment for integrated models of biomolecular interaction networks. Genome Research. 2003;**13**:2498-2504. DOI: 10.1101/gr.1239303

[61] Filippi CV, Aguirre N, Rivas JG, Zubrzycki J, Puebla A, Cordes D, et al. Population structure and genetic diversity characterization of a sunflower association mapping population using SSR and SNP markers. BMC Plant Biology. 2015;**15**:52. DOI: 10.1186/s12870-014-0360-x

[62] Gan S, Amasino RM. Making Sense of Senescence (Molecular Genetic Regulation and Manipulation of Leaf Senescence). Plant Physiology. 1997;**113**:313-319. Available: http://www.pubmedcentral.nih.gov/articlerender.fcgi?artid=158144<tool&pmcentrez&rendertype=abstract

[63] Hörtensteiner S. Chlorophyll degradation during senescence. Annual Review of Plant Biology. 2006;**57**:55-77

Chapter 4

Accelerated Senescence of Cancer Stem Cells: A Failure to Thrive or a Route to Survival?

Jekaterina Erenpreisa, Kristine Salmina and Mark Steven Cragg

Additional information is available at the end of the chapter

http://dx.doi.org/10.5772/intechopen.68582

Abstract

Accelerated senescence of cancer stem cells (CSCs) represents an adaptive response allowing withstand cell death. TP53, the pivotal tumor suppressor plays an important role in this process by inducing a prolonged dual state with senescence and self-renewal as potential outcomes. Molecularly, this is achieved by activating both OCT4A (POU5F1) and p21CIP1. OCT4A suppresses the excessive activity of p21 preventing the immediate precipitation of apoptosis or terminal senescence. It persists as long as sufficient cellular energy remains; generated through autophagy, itself sequestrating p16INK4A in the cytoplasm. As such, autophagic capacity is the bottleneck of these TP53-dependent senescence reversal processes, as well terminal senescence will follow if DNA damage is not ultimately repaired. In TP53 mutants the CSC-like state is boosted by stressed cells overcoming the tetraploidy barrier. These cells acquire additional DNA repair capacity through mitotic slippage and entrance to a sequence of ploidy cycles, allowing repair and sorting DNA damage, ultimately facilitating the genesis of mitotically competent daughter cells following final depolyploidisation. Again, autophagy is required to fuel this process. More detailed knowledge of these arcane processes anticipates the provision of anti-cancer drug targets, such as AURORA B kinase and Survivin, which ensure mitotic slippage and the continuity of ploidy cycles.

Keywords: accelerated senescence, cancer stem cells (CSCs), TP53, DNA damage, self-renewal OCT4A (POU5F1), p21CIP1, pluripotency, apoptosis, metastability, DNA repair, autophagy, p16INK4A, tetraploidy, ploidy cycles, AURORA B, Survivin, AMPK

1. Introduction

In 2001 Roninson and colleagues [1] published the now seminal article entitled "If not apoptosis, then what? Treatment-induced senescence and mitotic catastrophe in tumor cells". After decades of overwhelming attention toward apoptosis induction as the cure for cancer, this article gave birth to a new field in cancer research. They wrote: "Inhibition of the program of apoptosis has been reported to have little or no effect on clonogenic survival after treatment with drugs or radiation in several tumor cell lines. A decrease in apoptosis is compensated in such cell lines by an increase in the fractions of cells that undergo permanent growth arrest with phenotypic features of cell senescence. The senescent phenotype distinguishes tumor cells that survived drug exposure but lost the ability to form colonies from those that recover and proliferate after treatment. Although senescent cells do not proliferate, they are metabolically active and may produce secreted proteins with potential tumor-promoting activities."

Since that article, the induction of senescence was even claimed as the new goal of cancer treatment [2] and many researchers stepped on this path.

In this chapter, we describe our data over the last 2 decades, which along with other research, substantiates the exact opposite: that so-called accelerated cell senescence (ASC) (also called stress-induced premature senescence) and mitotic catastrophe (MC) are not desired goals of cancer treatment. Rather, we show that these processes can enable genotoxically treated cancer cells to escape cell death, not only by secretion of survival promoting components [3] but also by effective DNA repair. By stabilizing or recovering the innate stem properties of cancer stem cells (CSCs) senescence can be reversed by DNA damaged-induced ACS. To explore these concepts clearly it is first important to review and define the typical features of cell senescence and the biology of CSCs.

2. Biological features of cell senescence: what is clear and what is not?

Replicative senescence is usually dependent on *TP53*/p21CIP1/pRb/E2F pathway, whereas accelerated senescence can be mediated through *TP53*/p21CIP1/pRb/E2F or, p16ink4a/pRb/E2F pathway or both [4]. Cells acquire flat morphology, upregulate autophagy, and become positive for sa-β-galactosidase (pH 6.0) staining, indicative of high lysosomal activity. Erosion of telomeres and achievement of the Hayflick limit characterizes proliferative senescence, while in ACS the telomeres are not shortened [5]. However, the emergence of DNA strand breaks and the resulting DNA damage response (DDR) characterizes both proliferative and accelerated senescence [6]. Persistent irreparable DNA damage triggers the senescence-associated secretome [7], which is another feature of cell senescence. Emergence of endopolyploid cells, some capable of escaping senescence is also a typical feature of normal [8] and cancer cells [9, 10]. The reversibility of genotoxically induced senescence coupled to reversible polyploidy and its relation to stemness and population recovery are key phenomenon to understand if we wish to develop better cancer treatments [11–17]. The polyploidy component of senescence is associated with resistance to chemotherapy and involves mTOR activation; its inhibition causes senescence reversal, neo-expression of stem cell markers [18] and increased resistance of cancer cells to chemotherapy [19]. However, whether any senescing primary somatic cancer cell is capable of displaying the above features associated with senescence reversal or whether this only applies to cancer stem cells (CSCs) and how the recovery finally occurs is still largely unclear.

http://dx.doi.org/10.5772/intechopen.68582

3. The common biological features of embryonic stem cells (ESCs) and CSC

It is now generally accepted that CSCs play a central role in cancer genesis and promotion. Firstly, they possess the developmental potential, being capable of sphere formation and the ability to differentiate into mesoderm, endoderm and ectoderm progenies. Many gene modules of ESC are found active in various cancers [20], in turn, aggressive tumors express the markers of ESC or germ cells [21–24]. Third, tumors also acquire epigenetic profiles of ESC under genotoxic [25–28] or hypoxic conditions [29], in association with overcoming the tetraploidy barrier. So, epigenetically, CSCs of highly de-differentiated tumors possess many features of ESC.

Epigenetic instability is another notable feature of ESC and likely also of CSC. ESCs possess 'poised', chromatin marking of key developmental genes. Such marking consists of large regions of H3 lysine 27 methylation harboring smaller regions of H3 lysine 4 methylation. These domains tend to coincide with genes of transposable elements (TE) expressed at low levels [30]. Some activity of TE may provide the transcriptional noise, which is necessary for the fate changes observed during early embryo development [31, 32]. Moreover, the enhancers in ESCs are enriched for the transposable elements and genetic variations associated with cancer [33].

An additional peculiarity of ESC (and likewise CSC) is the absence of the cell cycle G1/S restriction checkpoint: here OCT4 and NANOG activate cyclin D kinases cdk4 and cdk6 [34] to force ESC into S-phase. Therefore, damaged ESC cells typically accumulate in the G2 DNA damage checkpoint instead, whose relative weakness allows mitotic slippage [35, 36]. Moreover, stressed ESC and likely also CSC possess a peculiar intermediate post-slippage phase (not 4 N-G1) [37, 38] containing non-degraded cyclin B1, which is normally destroyed after mitosis. In irradiated lymphomas and HeLa cells this nondegraded cyclin B1 was found to be sustained by activated Mos kinase [39]. Some additional activators of meiotic prophase were also revealed [40, 41] indicating a possible trigger from the mitotic DNA damage checkpoint into a meiotic prophase-like state with its more effective recombination checkpoint. Potentially, this meiosis-like molecular setting allows CSCs to tolerate both DNA damage and tetraploidy and use this compartment for DNA repair by homologous recombination [14, 42]. All three facets of CSC biology; poised chromatin, an epigenetic shift to embryonality, and the peculiar cell cycle checkpoints are apparently interrelated and involved in ACS, whose main hallmark is persistent DNA damage. The remainder of this chapter is an attempt to assess this notion within our experimental material.

4. Accelerated senescence of human fibroblasts induces senescing tetraploid cells with transient self-renewal potential

In one of our recent experimental systems, embryonal lung human fibroblasts (IMR90 cells) were grown in normoxia (20%) and 5% CO_2 and reached full senescence (proliferative arrest with zero mitotic index) after 32–34 passages. Senescence was characterized by flat morphology of enlarged cells, nuclear positivity of p21CIP1 and cytoplasmic accumulation of p16INK4A; at the terminally stage nuclei were swelling and p16 entered the cell nuclei [43]. DNA cytometry revealed an accumulation of a portion of the prematurely senescing cells in the G2 compartment (**Figure 1A, B**) which were also overcoming the tetraploidy barrier with formation of a few (4–6%) tetraploid cells, which sometimes entered aberrant mitoses. These cells with large polyploid nuclei began to express both senescence markers (p21CIP1 and p16INK4A) with the self-renewal marker NANOG; these cells were also positive for DNA double strand breaks (DSB) (**Figure 1C–F**). The acquisition of bi-potentiality by a small proportion of normal

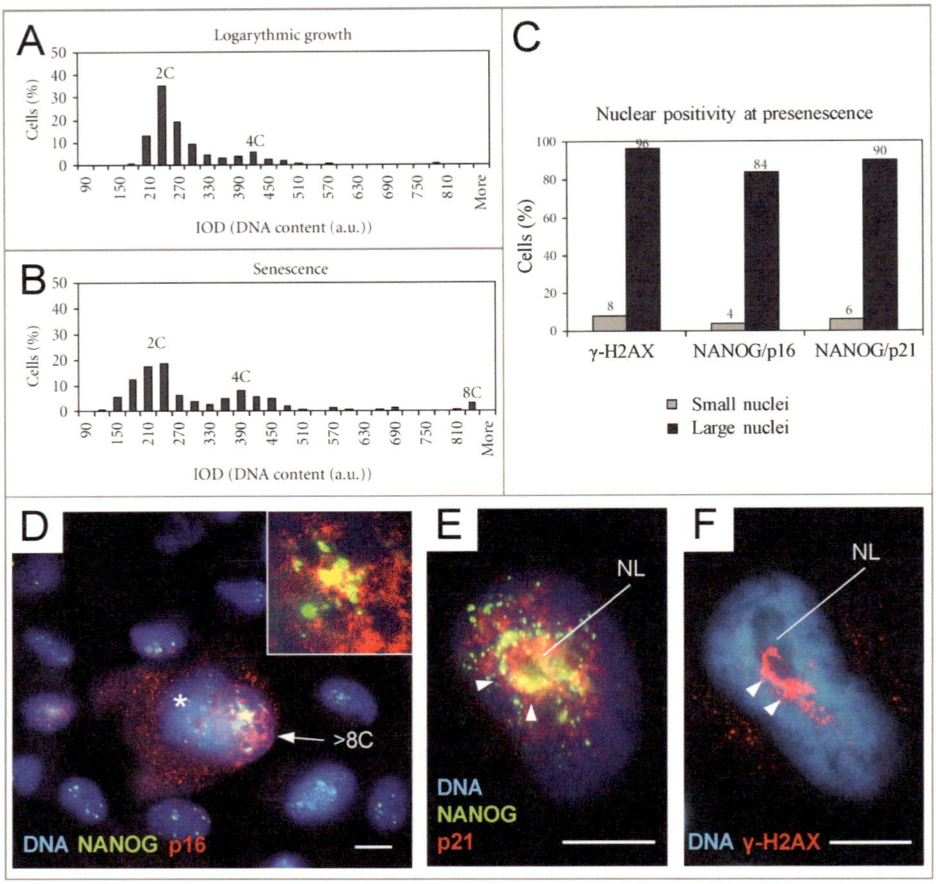

Figure 1. Characteristics of IMR90 human embryonal fibroblasts undergoing pre-senescence. Cells were cytospun, fixed and stained for DNA image cytometry. DNA content was determined for at least 200 cells in each condition and is represented as the percentage in a state of (**A**) logarithmic growth; (**B**) presenescence with some accumulation of cells in the G2M (4C) checkpoint and some increase of >4C DNA cell numbers. (**C**) shows the results from immunofluorescence studies staining for γ-H2AX, NANOG, P21CIP1 or p16INKA4A proteins with positive staining discriminated with respect to nuclei size; (**D–F**) – typical immunofluorescence patterns showing combinations of self-renewal (NANOG) and senescence (p21CIP1 and p16INK4A) markers in the same cells with large (>4C nuclei as measured by DAPI) nuclei, and positivity for DSBs γ-H2AX. Bars= 10 μm. Republished from Ref. [43].

cells overcoming the G2M DNA damage checkpoint is reminiscent of stem cell activity; with the same lack of arrest in the G1/S checkpoint and weak G2M checkpoint. Nevertheless, these cells did not persist in the culture and NANOG expression was lost in later passages.

These observations heightened our interest in the role of senescence in the CSC model.

5. Ovarian germline cells challenged by genotoxic stress display the dual p53-dependent expression of p21CIP1 and OCT4A

As a model for CSC we chose the ovarian germline cancer cells PA1. These cells are wt *TP53*, possessing features of embryonal carcinoma [44]. They were treated with etoposide (ETO), the inhibitor of Topoisomerase II, to induce DSB through the impairment of S-phase [45]. Cells entered massive, prolonged, G2-arrest, acquired flat morphology, and signaled persistent DDR for about 4–5 days in nearly 100% of cell nuclei (positive for γ-H2AX and CHK2 foci) with some cells overcoming the tetraploid barrier (**Figure 2A, B**). The most surprising fact was that regulators of the opposing processes of senescence (p21CIP1) and self-renewal OCT4A (POU5F1) were highly induced in the same G2-arrested cells (**Figures 2C** and **4A**). This was downstream of activated *TP53*, as both p21 and partly OCT4A became downregulated after *TP53* RNAi silencing (**Figure 2C**) [45]. Further study [46] revealed that p53-activated OCT4A down-regulated p21CIP1, moderating its expression and preventing cells from precipitating terminal senescence or apoptosis (**Figure 2D**), thus providing the opportunity for repair. Downregulation of p21 via OCT4 was previously shown in ESC [47].

Moreover, such stress-activated OCT4A was transiently disconnected from its self-renewal partners (SOX2 and NANOG), as those protein levels were low and/or not activated alongside Oct4A [46]. Therefore, the autoregulatory and feedforward loops seen in ESC [48] were not present, potentially due to the known down-regulation of the Nanog gene promoter by activated p53 [49] and/or the down-regulation of NANOG by high levels of OCT4A [50]. However, it is also possible that another, Cdk4-activating function of OCT4A [34] could be enhanced, while inhibiting action of p21on Cyclin D/cdk4,6 checkpoint function reduced forcing escape of the damaged cells from G1/S checkpoint leading to their accumulation in G2-arrest. **Figure 3** presents these hypothetical relationships between the cell cycle and pluripotency functions of stress-activated OCT4A induced by DNA damage through activated p53.

The bizarre duality of OCT4A with p21CIP1 was subdued and cell cycle in the PA1 clones returned to normal, on days 7–14 (**Figure 2A**), while silencing of stress-activated OCT4A prevented recovery [46]. This transient undecided state in G2 arrest, between true senescence and true self-renewal, was thus lasting as long as wt*TP53* was activated by the DNA DSB.

In accordance with our findings in PA1 cells after ETO treatment, a recent high-throughput RNAi screen revealed the intrinsic roles of S and G2, functionally establishing that pluripotency control is hardwired to the cell-cycle machinery and that the ATM/ATR-CHEK2-p53 axis enhances the TGF-b pathway to prevent premature cell death [36]. As well, [3] showed that

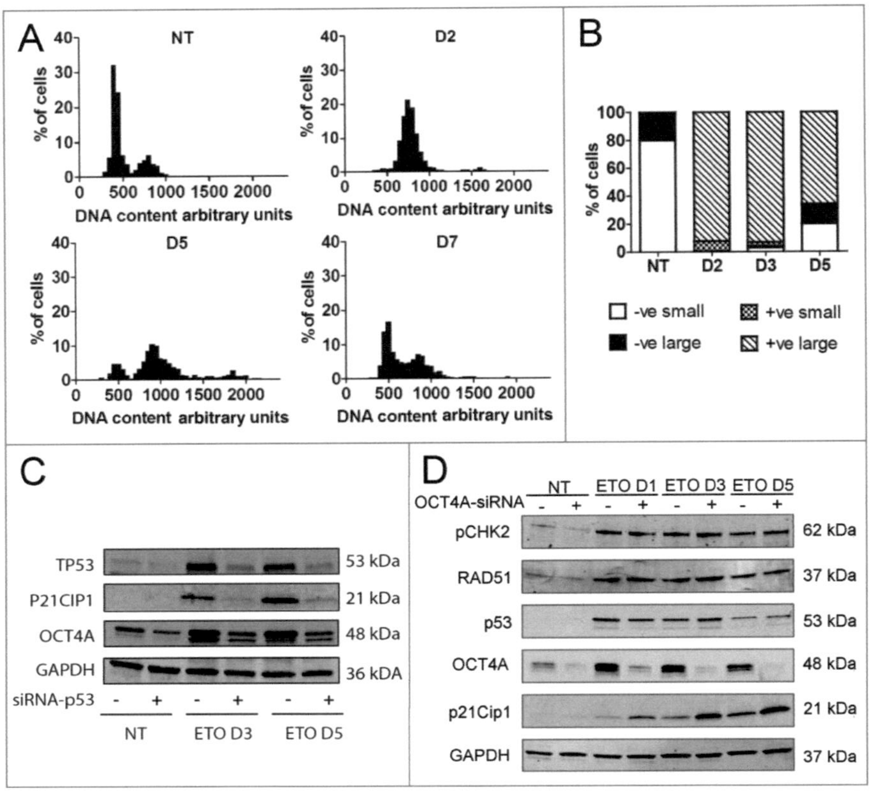

Figure 2. Response of PA -1 cells to ETO treatment. PA -1 cells were treated with 8 μM ETO for 20 h, then washed and assessed at the indicated time point. (**A**) Cells were cytospun, fixed and stained for DNA image cytometry as previously described [46]. DNA content was determined for at least 200 cells in each condition and is represented as a percentage. Profound G2 arrest on day 2 was observed followed by the simultaneous emergence of a polyploid (>4C) and 4nG1 fraction on day 5 before the recovery of the normal cell cycle profile by day 7. (**B**) The proportion of pCHK2-positive cells was examined in the context of DNA content with cells sub-divided into small or large cells. In the NT control sample, all cells were pCHK2-negative with an expected nuclei size distribution (2C 80%; ≥ 4C 20%). On day 2, all cells were pCHK2-positive and the vast majority of nuclei were large (≥4C). By day 5, cells with small nuclei appeared, all of which were pCHK2-negative. Data are representative of>three independent experiments; (**C**) Immunoblot analysis of TP53, OCT4A and P21CIP1 in PA-1 cells after ETO treatment. PA-1 cells were treated with non-target (ntg) siRNA (−) or siRNA-TP53 (+) for 24 h before treatment with 8 μM ETO, washing after 20 h and cell lysates made and assessed by immunoblotting for p53, P21CIP1, OCT4A or GAPDH as a loading control at the indicated time-points (day 3 and 5). p53 was upregulated in response to ETO treatment and suppressed by siRNA-*TP53*. P21CIP1 and OCT4A were also upregulated by ETO treatment, and the upregulation was restricted by treatment with siRNA-*TP53*. Data are representative of three independent experiments. (**A–C**) republished from Ref. [45]. (**D**) OCT4A suppresses p21CIP1 and induces senescence. PA-1 cells were treated with ntg-siRNA or OCT4-siRNA for 24 h before treatment with 8 μM ETO for 20 h and replacement with fresh media. Protein expression was assessed at the indicated time points by immunoblotting. Cell lysates were made and assessed by immunoblotting for pCHK2, RAD51, p53, p21CIP1, OCT4A and GAPDH as a loading control. Republished from Ref. [46].

cellular senescence accompanying DNA damage or DNA damage as such favors cell reprogramming in vivo models. It should be noted however, that the frequency (chance) of survival in our PA1-ETO model was not high. It stresses the importance of another possible player in this "undecided" stage between senescence and self-renewal, of transcriptional noise.

http://dx.doi.org/10.5772/intechopen.68582

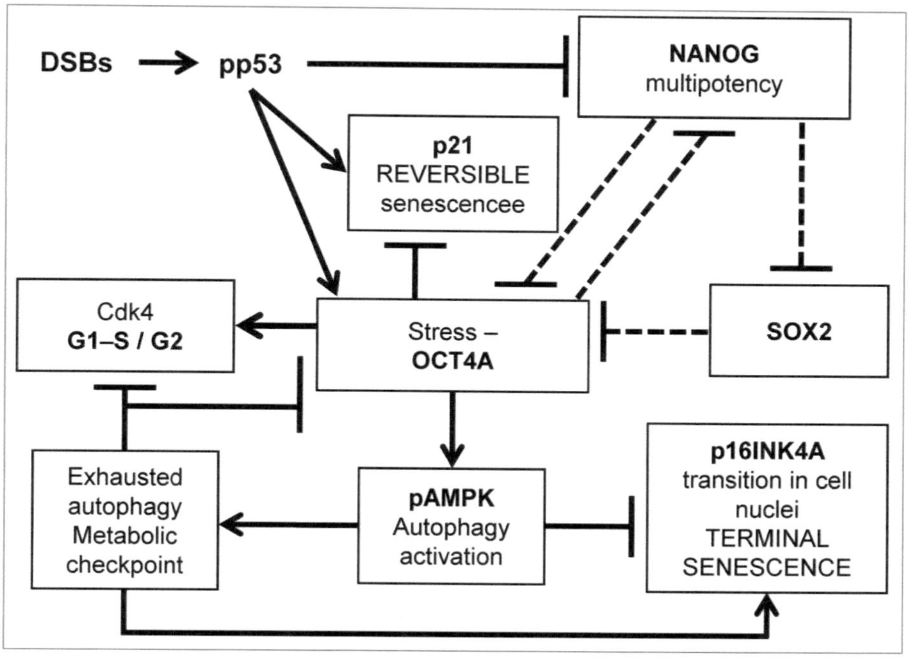

Figure 3. Schematic of the response of wt *TP53* cancer stem cells to genotoxic damage. P53 is activated and simultaneously induces p21CIP1 and OCT4A. OCT4A moderates the expression of p21CIP1 preventing apoptosis or terminal senescence [45, 46]. Activated p53 also downregulates the promoter of Nanog gene [49]. Therefore, the multipotency circuit based on Nanog stimulation of OCT4A and SOX2 [48] (dashed lines) is interrupted. In addition, the overexpressed OCT4A also down-regulates NANOG [50]. Activated OCT4A also enhances the activity of cdk4 and favors cells exit from the G1/S restriction checkpoint [34] and accumulation in G2. Activated p53 also activates pAMPK, likely via OCT4A. pAMPK activates autophagy. Functional autophagy sequesters and digests p16INKA4 within the cytoplasm, preventing its transition into the cell nuclei and hence terminal senescence. With exhaustion of autophagic capacity (halting of autophagic flux) pAMPK activates a metabolic checkpoint [51], which precipitates cell death in the G1 and possibly also G2 cell compartments.

6. Transient bi-potentiality of CSC for senescence and self-renewal displays the population features of "noisy" expression and activated transposable elements

One of the interesting facets of this dual expression of self-renewal and senescence regulators in the PA1-ETO model was the high heterogeneity in response, with individual cells expressing wildly differing levels of OCT4 and p21 (**Figure 4A**). This explorative chaos continued for 4–6 days and culminated with massive cell death selecting a small proportion (<1%) of resistant survivors. Earlier studies on ESC observing the extensive heterogeneity and fluctuations of gene expression in individual stem cells led the authors to suggest that "noise "may be the central driving force behind multipotency [32, 50, 52].

Therefore, notably, a similar long 'stochastic' phase of choice between senescence and self-renewal (initiated by activating DNA repair and mesenchymal to epithelial transition), with

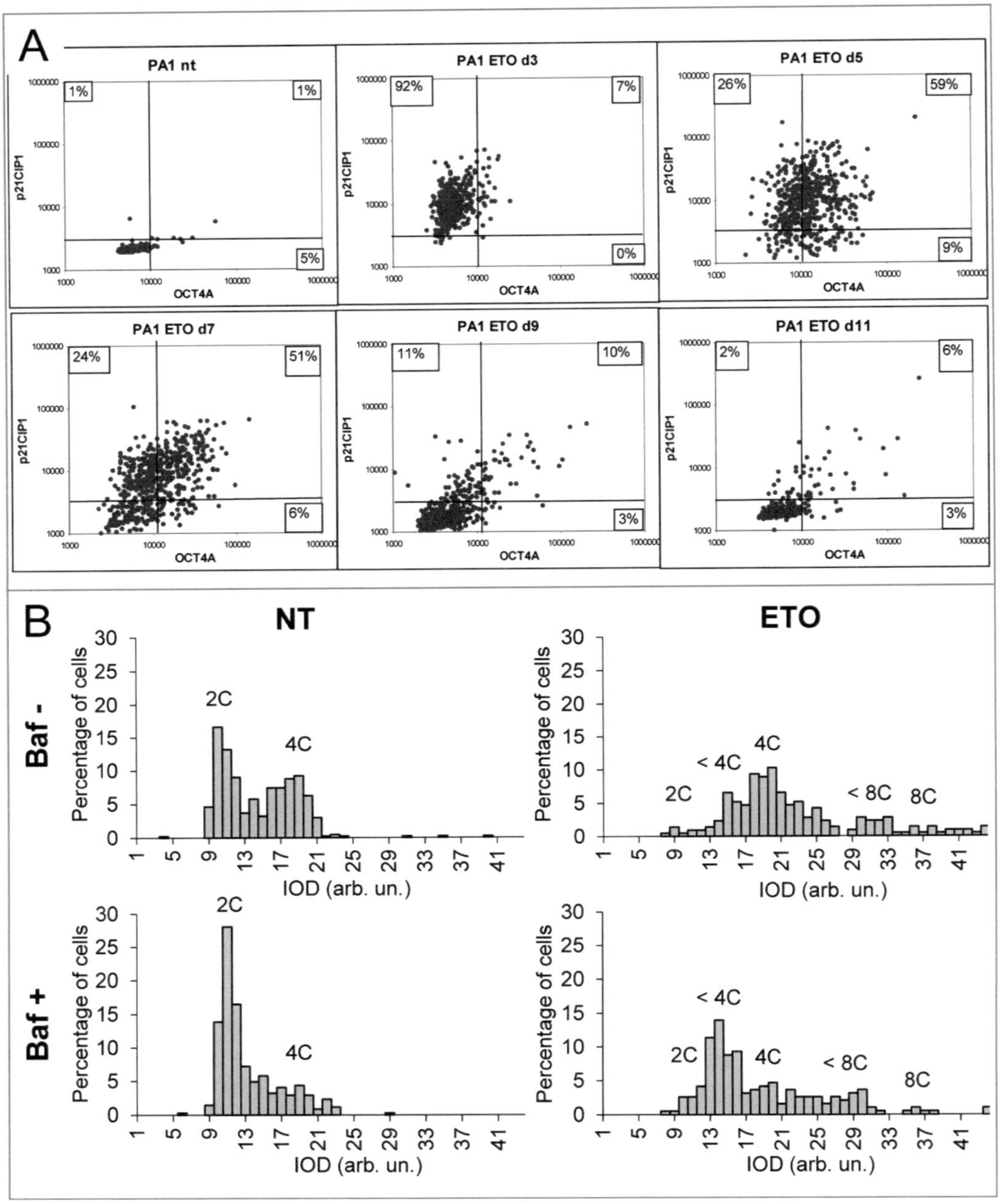

Figure 4. Population heterogeneity in expression of OCT4A and p21CIP1 in response of PA1 cells to ETO treatment. (**A**) Population heterogeneity in expression of OCT4A and p21CIP1 is extended for days 2–6 post ETO treatment, before recovery from day 7, when it reduces; (**B**) Population heterogeneity is accompanied by a degree of polyploidy as represented by DNA histograms on day 4, with underreplication of the cells in late S-phase of diploid and polyploid cell cohorts; this phenomenon is enhanced after impediment of autophagic flux. Republished from Ref. [46].

heterogenous activation of pluripotency genes, preceding the period of further determination of self-renewal circuitry has also been reported during the induction of pluripotent stem cells [53].

Our study of DNA histograms in ETO-treated PA1 cells revealed in addition to G2M arrest, a strong under-replication in late S-phase (**Figure 4B**), the time of constitutive heterochromatin replication [46]. Similarly, arrest in late S- and G2M phase was reported after Doxorubicin treatment in p53 mutant cancer cells [54]. This feature may therefore be equally required for any senescence causing release from silencing and subsequent activation of TE nested in constitutive heterochromatin as retrotransposition was found in replicative cell senescence [55, 56]. In particular, under-replication may cause de-repression of TE genes and result in the epigenetic activation of the developmental genes in the poised chromatin regions [30] enabling the reprogramming by senescence. Indeed, we observed the activation and clustering of *ALU* elements in the ETO treated PA1 cells [57]. The initial de-repression of transposons could provide the necessary "noisy" background of transcription allowing chaotic fluctuations of gene expression, which enable stochastic choice of the appropriate attractors for cell fate change and escape from terminal senescence.

7. The role of autophagy in preventing terminal senescence

Our further observations in the PA1 model showed the importance of autophagy in withstanding the proteotoxic stress following ETO treatment and its crucial role in maintaining viability; inhibition of autophagy culminated in chromatin fragmentation and nuclei disintegration [46, 57]. Stress-activated OCT4A mainly colocalized, and correlated in its nuclear concentration in individual cells, with activated AMP^{thr172} kinase (**Figure 5A, B**). AMP-activated protein kinase (AMPK) serves as a general energy depletion sensor and activator of autophagy. The energy stress-response of AMPK is also tightly linked to the DDR of p53 [58, 59] and can induce a p53-dependent glucose-sensitive metabolic checkpoint [51] precipitating apoptotic cell death from the G1/S and likely autophagic death from G2M checkpoint [60].

We found, in addition, that active autophagy in PA1-ETO cells sequestered p16INK4A aggresomes within the autophagic vacuoles (**Figure 5C** i–ii), while disability of autophagy enabled p16 diffuse distribution in the cell nuclei and caused terminal senescence with nuclear disintegration (**Figure 5** iii-iv) preventing survival of ETO-treated cells [46]. The p53-dependent role of AMPK, its relationship with stress-activated OCT4A, and the role of autophagy in the prevention of terminal senescence for TP53 wild-type CSC cells is schematically presented in **Figure 3**.

However, in *TP53* mutants, the cells find an additional pathway for potential recovery – they undergo mitotic slippage and employ polyploidy for repair and sorting the damaged DNA.

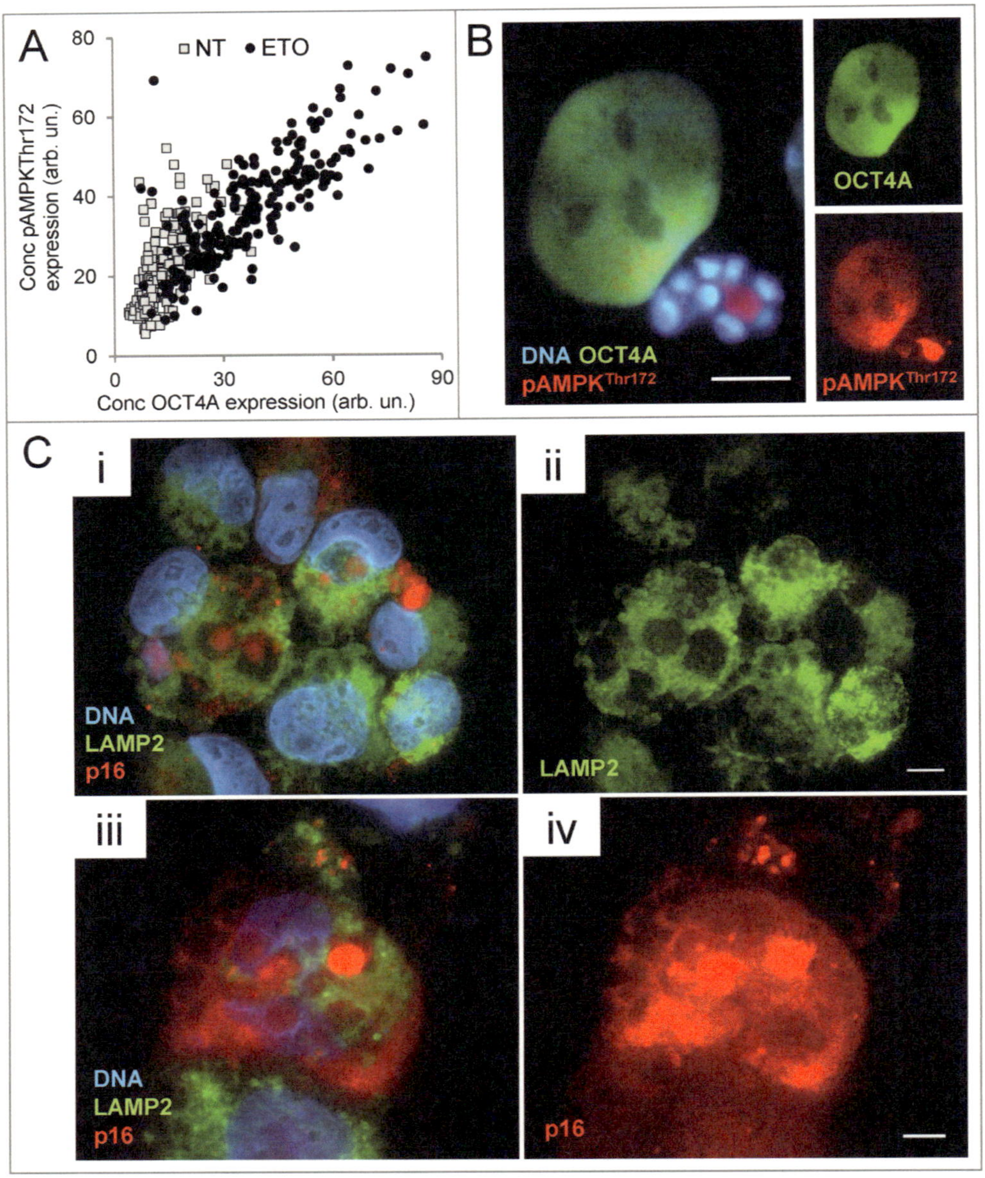

Figure 5. Autophagic response of PA1 cells to ETO-mediated DNA damage: (**A**) Scatterplot of image cytometry of OCT4A and pAMPK in individual cells assessed on day 4 after ETO treatment. There is a clear correlation between enhanced expression of OCT4A and $pAMPK^{Thr172}$ of ETO-treated cells; (**B**) OCT4A and $pAMPK^{Thr172}$ immunofluorescence in PA-1 cells 4 days after ETO-treatment. (**C**) The relationship between autophagy and senescence. PA1-ETO cells were treated without or with Bafilomycin A1, prior to media being removed and replaced with fresh media; cells were harvested 48 h later (day 4). (i) imunofluorescent staining for p16ink4a, LAMP2 or DAPI as shown via the BRG optical filter, (ii) only LAMP2 demonstrating high level of functional autophagy sequestrating p16ink4a-containing aggresomes. (iii–iv) shows an example of autophagic failure, where sequestration of p16ink4a is partly lost, diffusing into the cytoplasm and nucleus, which is destroyed. Bars = 10 μm. Republished from Ref. [46].

8. *TP53* mutants with persistent DNA damage undergo mitotic slippage, ploidy cycles, and are capable of reversing senescence alongside polyploidy

Some authors have reported that genotoxically treated cancer cells can paradoxically combine sa-β-gal-positivity (considered as a universal marker of senescence) with expression of Ki67, a hallmark signature of proliferation. This "swing phenotype" is apparently dependent on p21 and TERT [61]. Others have reported that sa-β-gal-positivity is also compatible with polylploid cells (induced by DNA chemotherapy) undergoing de-polyploidization and surviving [13, 16]. Overcoming the tetraploidy barrier in *TP53* mutants, boosting the self-renewal network [25, 26] – can likely convert tumor cells into CSCs or stabilize them. Moreover, paradoxically, genotoxically challenged *TP53* mutant tumor cells, which uncouple DNA replication from cell division and undergo mitotic slippage possessing both DNA DSBs and Ki67 expression (**Figure 6A**). As well the mitotic chromo-

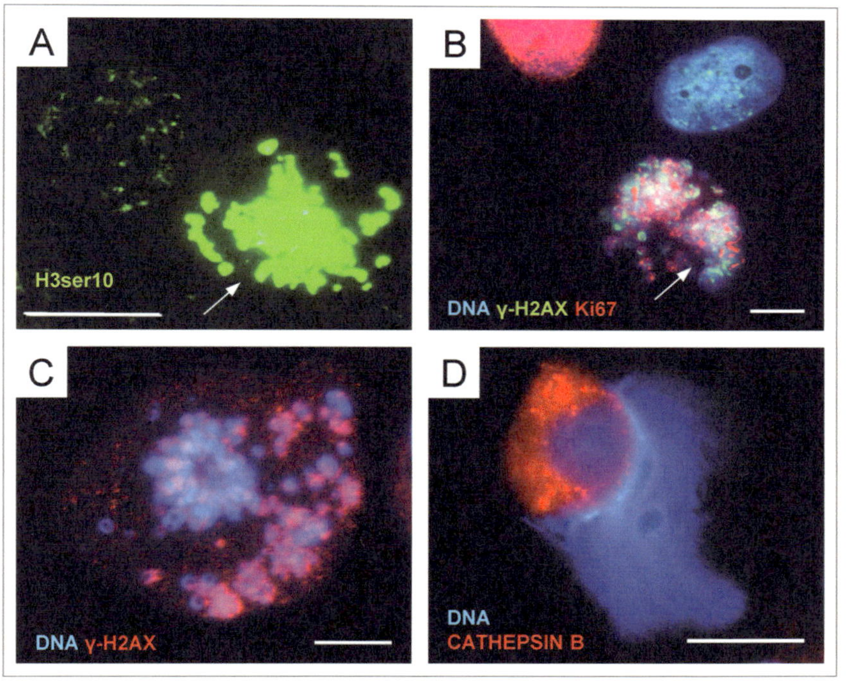

Figure 6. Mutant *TP53* tumors have additional options for repair and sorting of DNA damage in ploidy cycles. The genotoxic damage in mutant TP53 cancer cell lines of various origins favors mitotic slippage with exaggerated: (**A**) H3ser10 activation by mitotic AURBK and (**B**) expression of proliferation marker Ki67 tolerating DNA damage detected by γ-H2AX foci. This is followed by (**C**) DNA damage sorting by micronuclei in the next mitosis of the polyploid cells and/or (**D**) by expelling and autophagic digestion of the whole subnuclei of multi-nucleated cells. (**A**) HeLa cells, 10 Gy irradiation, day 4; (**B**) MDA MB 231 breast cancer cells on day 4 after 100nM Doxorubicin treatment (in collaboration with A. Boiko); (**C**) SK-Mel-28 cell, 30Gy, day 2 (in collaboration with TR Jackson); (**D**) WI-L2-NS lymphoblastoma, 10Gy, day 6. Republished from Ref. [62]. Bars (A)=20 μm; (B–D)=10 μm.

some passengers, such as catalytically active Aurora B kinase (**Figure 6B**) and Survivin are expressed during mitotic slippage and in resulting polyploidy interphase [19, 63, 64]. Notably, activated AMPK, responsible for the metabolic aspect of senescence-associated autophagy, also possesses these same chromosome passenger features [65]. All of these observations indicate that stress-induced "senescent" cancer cells retain their proliferation potential through induced polyploidy coupled to active autophagy. During this process or/and in the next tetraploid/octaploid cell cycle they can additionally repair DNA [42] and also sort the un-repaired DNA damage in micronuclei (**Figure 6C**), as first reported by Haaf et al. [66]. The autophagic nature of this sorting found by Rello-Varona et al. [67]; has been reviewed previously in Ref. [68]. This sorting of the DNA damage through micronucleation was observed by us in several tumor cell line models after different kinds of genotoxic treatments as exemplified in **Figure 6 (A–C)**. The autophagic elimination of large DNA portions or whole sub-nuclei with damaged DNA was also observed (**Figure 6D**) [62, 68, 69] as another intriguing feature of the late post-damage events of genotoxically treated *TP53* mutants.

All this indicates that *TP53* mutants have a strong capacity for surviving genotoxic damage and reversing cell senescence by reversible endopolyploidy through a pathway involving boosted stemness. This pathway is in fact far away from the regulations of the typical mammalian cell cycle. More likely, these tumor cells exploit the life-cycle-like regulations of the unicellular organisms recapitulated from evolutionary ploidy cycles as we have postulated previously in Refs. [70, 71] and showed recently by bioinformatics study of polyploidy [72]. It only remains to add that in general tumor cells cannot bear wild type *TP53* and inactivate it, if not by mutations, then in many other ways [73]. Perhaps the increased ability to access additional routes to cell survival by overcoming senescence and repairing DNA damage as detailed above, also help explain this inactivation of *TP53* function in tumors.

Acknowledgements

Mr. Jekabs Krigerts is acknowledged for formatting the article and illustrations.

Author details

Jekaterina Erenpreisa[1]*, Kristine Salmina[1] and Mark Steven Cragg[2]

*Address all correspondence to: katrina@biomed.lu.lv

1 Tumour Cell Biology Group, Latvian Biomedical Research and Study Centre, Riga, Latvia

2 Antibody and Vaccine Group, Cancer Sciences Unit, Faculty of Medicine, General Hospital, University of Southampton, Southampton, United Kingdom

References

[1] Roninson IB, Broude EV., Chang BD. If not apoptosis, then what? Treatment-induced senescence and mitotic catastrophe in tumor cells. Drug Resistance Updates. 2001;**4**(5):303-313. DOI: 10.1054/drup.2001.0213

[2] Shay JW, Roninson IB. Hallmarks of senescence in carcinogenesis and cancer therapy. Oncogene. 2004;**23**(16):2919-2933. DOI: 10.1038/sj.onc.1207518

[3] Mosteiro L, Pantoja C, Alcazar N, Marión RM, Chondronasiou D, Rovira M, et al. Tissue damage and senescence provide critical signals for cellular reprogramming in vivo. Science (80-). 2016;**354**(6315):aaf4445. DOI: 10.1126/science.aaf4445

[4] Collado M, Blasco MA, Serrano M. Cellular senescence in cancer and aging. Cell. 2007;**130**(2):223-233. DOI: 10.1016/j.cell.2007.07.003

[5] Suzuki M, Boothman DA. Stress-induced premature senescence (SIPS)–influence of SIPS on radiotherapy. Journal of Radiation Research. 2008;**49**(2):105-112

[6] d'Adda di Fagagna F. Living on a break: Cellular senescence as a DNA-damage response. Nature Reviews Cancer. 2008;**8**(7):512-522. DOI: 10.1038/nrc2440

[7] Rodier F, Coppé JP, Patil CK, Hoeijmakers WAM, Muñoz DP, Raza SR, et al. Persistent DNA damage signalling triggers senescence-associated inflammatory cytokine secretion. Nature Cell Biology. 2009;**11**(8):973-979. DOI: 10.1038/ncb1909

[8] Walen KH. Human diploid fibroblast cells in senescence; cycling through polyploidy to mitotic cells. In Vitro Cellular & Developmental Biology: Animal. 2006;**42**(7):216-224. DOI: 10.1290/0603019.1

[9] Mosieniak G, Sikora E. Polyploidy: The link between senescence and cancer. Current Pharmaceutical Design. 2010;**16**(6):734-740

[10] Mosieniak G, Sliwinska MA, Alster O, Strzeszewska A, Sunderland P, Piechota M, et al. Polyploidy formation in doxorubicin-treated cancer cells can favor escape from senescence. Neoplasia. 2015;**17**(12):882-893. DOI: 10.1016/j.neo.2015.11.008

[11] Sundaram M, Guernsey DL, Rajaraman MM, Rajaraman R. Neosis: A novel type of cell division in cancer. Cancer Biology and Therapy. 2004;**3**(2):207-218

[12] Tam WL, Ang YS, Lim B. The molecular basis of ageing in stem cells. Mechanisms of Ageing and Development. 2007;**128**(1):137-148. DOI: 10.1016/j.mad.2006.11.020

[13] Puig PE, Guilly MN, Bouchot A, Droin N, Cathelin D, Bouyer F, et al. Tumor cells can escape DNA-damaging cisplatin through DNA endoreduplication and reversible polyploidy. Cell Biology International. 2008;**32**(9):1031-1043. DOI: 10.1016/j.cellbi.2008.04.021

[14] Erenpreisa J, Cragg MS. Three steps to the immortality of cancer cells: Senescence, polyploidy and self-renewal. Cancer Cell International. 2013;**13**(1):92. DOI: 10.1186/1475-2867-13-92

[15] Wang Q, Wu PC, Dong DZ, Ivanova I, Chu E, Zeliadt S, et al. Polyploidy road to therapy-induced cellular senescence and escape. International Journal of Cancer. 2013;**132**(7):1505-1515. DOI: 10.1002/ijc.27810

[16] Sikora E, Mosieniak G, Sliwinska MA. Morphological and functional characteristic of senescent cancer cells. Current Drug Targets. 2016;**17**(4):377-387

[17] Sabisz M, Skladanowski A. Cancer stem cells and escape from drug-induced premature senescence in human lung tumor cells: Implications for drug resistance and in vitro drug screening models. Cell Cycle. 2009;**8**(19):3208-3217. DOI: 10.4161/cc.8.19.9758

[18] Chitikova Z V, Gordeev SA, Bykova TV, Zubova SG, Pospelov VA, Pospelova TV. Sustained activation of DNA damage response in irradiated apoptosis-resistant cells induces reversible senescence associated with mTOR downregulation and expression of stem cell markers. Cell Cycle. 2014;**13**(9):1424-1439. DOI: 10.4161/cc.28402

[19] Sharma S, Yao HP, Zhou YQ, Zhou J, Zhang R, Wang MH. Prevention of BMS-777607-induced polyploidy/senescence by mTOR inhibitor AZD8055 sensitizes breast cancer cells to cytotoxic chemotherapeutics. Molecular Oncology. 2014;**8**(3):469-482. DOI: 10.1016/j.molonc.2013.12.014

[20] Wong DJ, Liu H, Ridky TW, Cassarino D, Segal E, Chang HY. Module map of stem cell genes guides creation of epithelial cancer stem cells. Cell Stem Cell. 2008;**2**(4):333-344. DOI: 10.1016/j.stem.2008.02.009

[21] Old LJ. Cancer/testis (CT) antigens – A new link between gametogenesis and cancer. Cancer Immunity. 2001;**1**:1

[22] Kalejs M, Erenpreisa J. Cancer/testis antigens and gametogenesis: A review and "brain-storming" session. Cancer Cell International. 2005;**5**(1):4. DOI: 10.1186/1475-2867-5-4

[23] Kalejs M, Ivanov A, Plakhins G, Cragg MS, Emzinsh D, Illidge TM, et al. Upregulation of meiosis-specific genes in lymphoma cell lines following genotoxic insult and induction of mitotic catastrophe. BMC Cancer. 2006;**6**(1):6. DOI: 10.1186/1471-2407-6-6

[24] Ben-Porath I, Thomson MW, Carey VJ, Ge R, Bell GW, Regev A, et al. An embryonic stem cell-like gene expression signature in poorly differentiated aggressive human tumors. Nature Genetics. 2008;**40**(5):499-507. DOI: 10.1038/ng.127

[25] Salmina K, Jankevics E, Huna A, Perminov D, Radovica I, Klymenko T, et al. Up-regulation of the embryonic self-renewal network through reversible polyploidy in irradiated p53-mutant tumour cells. Experimental Cell Research. 2010;**316**(13):2099-2112. DOI: 10.1016/j.yexcr.2010.04.030

[26] Lagadec C, Vlashi E, Della Donna L, Dekmezian C, Pajonk F. Radiation-induced reprogramming of breast cancer cells. Stem Cells. 2012;**30**(5):833-844. DOI: 10.1002/stem.1058

[27] Vlashi E, Pajonk F. Cancer stem cells, cancer cell plasticity and radiation therapy. Seminars in Cancer Biology 2015;**31**:28-35. DOI: 10.1016/j.semcancer.2014.07.001

[28] Gerashchenko BI, Salmina K, Eglitis J, Huna A, Grjunberga V, Erenpreisa J. Disentangling the aneuploidy and senescence paradoxes: A study of triploid breast cancers non-responsive to neoadjuvant therapy. Histochemistry and Cell Biology. 2016;**145**(4):497-508. DOI: 10.1007/s00418-016-1415-x

[29] Zhang S, Mercado-Uribe I, Xing Z, Sun B, Kuang J, Liu J. Generation of cancer stem-like cells through the formation of polyploid giant cancer cells. Oncogene. 2014;**33**(1):116-128. DOI: 10.1038/onc.2013.96

[30] Bernstein BE, Mikkelsen TS, Xie X, Kamal M, Huebert DJ, Cuff J, et al. A bivalent chromatin structure marks key developmental genes in embryonic stem cells. Cell. 2006;**125**(2):315-326. DOI: 10.1016/j.cell.2006.02.041

[31] Peaston AE, Knowles BB, Hutchison KW. Genome plasticity in the mouse oocyte and early embryo. Biochemical Society Transactions. 2007;**35**(3):618-622. DOI: 10.1042/BST0350618

[32] Chang HH, Hemberg M, Barahona M, Ingber DE, Huang S. Transcriptome-wide noise controls lineage choice in mammalian progenitor cells. Nature. 2008;**453**(7194):544-547. DOI: 10.1038/nature06965

[33] Teng L, He B, Gao P, Gao L, Tan K. Discover context-specific combinatorial transcription factor interactions by integrating diverse ChIP-Seq data sets. Nucleic Acids Research. 2014;**42**(4):e24. DOI: 10.1093/nar/gkt1105

[34] Neganova I, Lako M. G1 to S phase cell cycle transition in somatic and embryonic stem cells. Journal of Anatomy. 2008;**213**(1):30-44. DOI: 10.1111/j.1469-7580.2008.00931.x

[35] Boheler KR. Stem cell pluripotency: A cellular trait that depends on transcription factors, chromatin state and a checkpoint deficient cell cycle. Journal of Cellular Physiology. 2009;**221**(1):10-17. DOI: 10.1002/jcp.21866

[36] Gonzales KAU, Liang H, Lim YS, Chan YS, Yeo JC, Tan CP, et al. Deterministic restriction on pluripotent state dissolution by cell-cycle pathways. Cell. 2015;**162**(3):564-579. DOI: 10.1016/j.cell.2015.07.001

[37] Mantel C, Guo Y, Lee MR, Kim MK, Han MK, Shibayama H, et al. Checkpoint-apoptosis uncoupling in human and mouse embryonic stem cells: A source of karyotpic instability. Blood. 2007;**109**(10):4518-4527. DOI: 10.1182/blood-2006-10-054247

[38] Mantel C, Guo Y, Lee MR, Han MK, Rhorabough S, Kim KS, et al. Cells enter a unique intermediate 4 N stage, not 4 N-G1, after aborted mitosis. Cell Cycle. 2008;**7**(4):484-492. DOI: 10.4161/cc.7.4.5316

[39] Erenpreisa J, Kalejs M, Cragg M. Mitotic catastrophe and endomitosis in tumour cells: An evolutionary key to a molecular solution. Cell Biology International. 2005;29(12):1012-1018. DOI: 10.1016/j.cellbi.2005.10.005

[40] Ianzini F, Kosmacek EA, Nelson ES, Napoli E, Erenpreisa J, Kalejs M, et al. Activation of meiosis-specific genes is associated with depolyploidization of human tumor cells following radiation-induced mitotic catastrophe. Cancer Research. 2009;**69**(6):2296-2304. DOI: 10.1158/0008-5472.CAN-08-3364

[41] Erenpreisa J, Cragg MS, Salmina K, Hausmann M, Scherthan H. The role of meiotic cohesin REC8 in chromosome segregation in gamma irradiation-induced endopolyploid tumour cells. Experimental Cell Research. 2009;**315**(15):2593-2603. DOI: 10.1016/j.yexcr.2009.05.011

[42] Ivanov A, Cragg MS, Erenpreisa J, Emzinsh D, Lukman H, Illidge TM. Endopolyploid cells produced after severe genotoxic damage have the potential to repair DNA double strand breaks. Journal of Cell Science. 2003;**116**(20):4095-4106. DOI: 10.1242/jcs.00740

[43] Huna A, Salmina K, Jascenko E, Duburs G, Inashkina I, Erenpreisa J. Self-renewal signalling in presenescent tetraploid IMR90 cells. Journal of Aging Research 2011;**2011**:103253. DOI: 10.4061/2011/103253

[44] Lifantseva N, Koltsova A, Krylova T, Yakovleva T, Poljanskaya G, Gordeeva O. Expression patterns of cancer-testis antigens in human embryonic stem cells and their cell derivatives indicate lineage tracks. Stem Cells International 2011;**2011**:1-13. DOI: 10.4061/2011/795239

[45] Jackson TR, Salmina K, Huna A, Inashkina I, Jankevics E, Riekstina U, et al. DNA damage causes TP53-dependent coupling of self-renewal and senescence pathways in embryonal carcinoma cells. Cell Cycle. 2013;**12**(3):430-441. DOI: 10.4161/cc.23285

[46] Huna A, Salmina K, Erenpreisa J, Vazquez-Martin A, Krigerts J, Inashkina I, et al. Role of stress-activated OCT4A in the cell fate decisions of embryonal carcinoma cells treated with etoposide. Cell Cycle. 2015;**14**(18):2969-2984. DOI: 10.1080/15384101.2015.1056948

[47] Lee J, Go Y, Kang I, Han YM, Kim J. Oct-4 controls cell-cycle progression of embryonic stem cells. The Biochemical Journal. 2010;**426**(2):171-181. DOI: 10.1042/BJ20091439

[48] Boyer LA, Lee TI, Cole MF, Johnstone SE, Levine SS, Zucker JP, et al. Core transcriptional regulatory circuitry in human embryonic stem cells. Cell. 2005;**122**(6):947-956. DOI: 10.1016/j.cell.2005.08.020

[49] Lin T, Chao C, Saito S, Mazur SJ, Murphy ME, Appella E, et al. p53 induces differentiation of mouse embryonic stem cells by suppressing Nanog expression. Nature Cell Biology. 2005;**7**(2):165-171. DOI: 10.1038/ncb1211

[50] Kalmar T, Lim C, Hayward P, Muñoz-Descalzo S, Nichols J, Garcia-Ojalvo J, et al. Regulated fluctuations in nanog expression mediate cell fate decisions in embryonic stem cells. Goodell MA, editor. PLoS Biology. 2009;**7**(7):e1000149. DOI: 10.1371/journal.pbio.1000149

[51] Jones RG, Plas DR, Kubek S, Buzzai M, Mu J, Xu Y, et al. AMP-activated protein kinase induces a p53-dependent metabolic checkpoint. Molecular Cell. 2005;**18**(3):283-293. DOI: 10.1016/j.molcel.2005.03.027

[52] Huang S, Eichler G, Bar-Yam Y, Ingber DE. Cell fates as high-dimensional attractor states of a complex gene regulatory network. Physical Reviews Letters. 2005;**94**(12):128701. DOI: 10.1103/PhysRevLett.94.128701

[53] Buganim Y, Faddah DA, Jaenisch R. Mechanisms and models of somatic cell reprogramming. Nature Reviews. Genetics.. 2013;**14**(6):427-439. DOI: 10.1038/nrg3473

[54] Shin HJ, Kwon HK, Lee JH, Gui X, Achek A, Kim JH, et al. Doxorubicin-induced necrosis is mediated by poly-(ADP-ribose) polymerase 1 (PARP1) but is independent of p53. Scientific Reports. 2015;**5**:15798. DOI: 10.1038/srep15798

[55] De Cecco M, Criscione SW, Peckham EJ, Hillenmeyer S, Hamm EA, Manivannan J, et al. Genomes of replicatively senescent cells undergo global epigenetic changes leading to gene silencing and activation of transposable elements. Aging Cell. 2013;**12**(2):247-256. DOI: 10.1111/acel.12047

[56] Sturm Á, Ivics Z, Vellai T. The mechanism of ageing: Primary role of transposable elements in genome disintegration. Cellular and Molecular Life Sciences. 2015;**72**(10):1839-1847. DOI: 10.1007/s00018-015-1896-0

[57] Salmina K, Huna A, Inashkina I, Belyayev A, Krigerts J, Pastova L, et al. Nucleolar aggresomes mediate release of pericentric heterochromatin and nuclear destruction of genotoxically treated cancer cells. Nucleus. 2017;**8**(2):205-221. DOI: 10.1080/19491034.2017.1279775

[58] Vazquez-Martin A, Oliveras-Ferraros C, Cufí S, Martin-Castillo B, Menendez JA. Metformin activates an Ataxia Telangiectasia Mutated (ATM)/Chk2-regulated DNA damage-like response. Cell Cycle. 2011;**10**(9):1499-1501. DOI: 10.4161/cc.10.9.15423

[59] Bungard D, Fuerth BJ, Zeng PY, Faubert B, Maas NL, Viollet B, et al. Signaling kinase AMPK activates stress-promoted transcription via histone H2B phosphorylation. Science (80-). 2010;**329**(5996):1201-1205. DOI: 10.1126/science.1191241

[60] Law BYK, Gordillo-Martínez F, Qu QY, Zhang N, Xu WS, Cogh PS, et al. Thalidezine, a novel AMPK activator, eliminates apoptosis - resistant cancer cells through energy-mediated autophagic cell death. Oncotarget. 2017

[61] Sherman MY, Meng L, Stampfer M, Gabai VL, Yaglom JA. Oncogenes induce senescence with incomplete growth arrest and suppress the DNA damage response in immortalized cells. Aging Cell. 2011;**10**(6):949-961. DOI: 10.1111/j.1474-9726.2011.00736.x

[62] Erenpreisa J, Salmina K, Huna A, Kosmacek EA, Cragg MS, Ianzini F, et al. Polyploid tumour cells elicit paradiploid progeny through depolyploidizing divisions and regulated autophagic degradation. Cell Biol Int. 2011;**35**(7):687-95. DOI: 10.1042/CBI20100762

[63] Erenpreisa J, Ivanov A, Wheatley SP, Kosmacek EA, Ianzini F, Anisimov AP, et al. Endopolyploidy in irradiated p53-deficient tumour cell lines: Persistence of cell division activity in giant cells expressing Aurora-B kinase. Cell Biology International. 2008;**32**(9):1044-1056. DOI: 10.1016/j.cellbi.2008.06.003

[64] Unruhe B, Schroder E, Wunsch D, Knauer SK. An old flame never dies: Survivin in cancer and cellular senescence. Gerontology. 2015;**62**(2):173-181. DOI: 10.1159/000432398

[65] Vazquez-Martin A, Oliveras-Ferraros C, Menendez JA. The active form of the metabolic sensor AMP-activated protein kinase α (AMPKα) directly binds the mitotic apparatus and travels from centrosomes to the spindle midzone during mitosis and cytokinesis. Cell Cycle. 2009;**8**(15):2385-2398. DOI: 10.4161/cc.8.15.9082

[66] Haaf T, Raderschall E, Reddy G, Ward DC, Radding CM, Golub EI. Sequestration of mammalian Rad51-recombination protein into micronuclei. The Journal of Cell Biology. 1999;**144**(1):11-20

[67] Rello-Varona S, Lissa D, Shen S, Niso-Santano M, Senovilla L, Mariño G, et al. Autophagic removal of micronuclei. Cell Cycle. 2012;**11**(1):170-176. DOI: 10.4161/cc.11.1.18564

[68] Erenpreisa J, Huna A, Salmina K, Jackson TR, Cragg MS. Macroautophagy-aided elimination of chromatin: Sorting of waste, sorting of fate? Autophagy. 2012;**8**(12):1877-1881

[69] Erenpreisa JA, Cragg MS, Fringes B, Sharakhov I, Illidge TM. Release of mitotic descendants by giant cells from irradiated Burkitt's lymphoma cell line. Cell Biology International. 2000;**24**(9):635-648. DOI: 10.1006/cbir.2000.0558

[70] Erenpreisa J, Cragg MS. Cancer: A matter of life cycle? Cell Biology International. 2007;**31**(12):1507-1510. DOI: 10.1016/j.cellbi.2007.08.013

[71] Erenpreisa J, Cragg MS. Life-cycle features of tumour cells. In: Pontarotti P, editor. Evolutionary Biology from Concept to Application. Berlin, Heidelberg: Springer Berlin Heidelberg; 2008. pp. 61-71. DOI: 10.1007/978-3-540-78993-2_4

[72] Vazquez-Martin A, Anatskaya OV, Giuliani A, Erenpreisa J, Huang S, Salmina K, et al. Somatic polyploidy is associated with the upregulation of c-MYC interacting genes and EMT-like signature. Oncotarget. 2016;**7**(46):75235-75260. DOI: 10.18632/oncotarget.12118

[73] Kastan MB. Wild-type p53: Tumors can't stand it. Cell. 2007;**128**(5):837-840. DOI: 10.1016/j.cell.2007.02.022

Chapter 5

Aging and Neurological Diseases

Marta Kowalska, Michal Owecki, Michal Prendecki,
Katarzyna Wize, Joanna Nowakowska,
Wojciech Kozubski, Margarita Lianeri and
Jolanta Dorszewska

Additional information is available at the end of the chapter

http://dx.doi.org/10.5772/intechopen.69499

Abstract

Current knowledge indicates that the aging process starts with subclinical changes at the molecular level. These include the accumulation of mutations, telomere attrition, and epigenetic alterations leading to genomic instability. Such defects multiply exponentially over time, resembling a "snowball effect," and eventually leading to morphological and functional deterioration of the brain, including progressive neuronal loss, reduced levels of neurotransmitters, excessive inflammation, and disrupted integrity of vessels, followed by infarction and microbleeds. Additionally, the decreasing efficiency of DNA repair mechanisms increases the susceptibility to reactive oxygen species and spontaneous mutagenesis, resulting in age-related neoplasia. Moreover, the malnutrition and malabsorption seen commonly in the elderly may cause deficiency of vitamin B_{12} and folic acid, both necessary for homocysteine metabolism, and lead to vascular damage. Altogether, these lead to brain damage in old age and greatly increase the risk of developing diseases of the central nervous system, such as stroke, epilepsy, Parkinson's disease, Alzheimer's disease, and other dementias.

Keywords: aging, molecular factor, neurological diseases

1. Introduction

Physiological aging starts after 60 years of age. Senescence in both animal models and humans is accompanied by alterations in the function of central cholinergic neurons. These changes essentially involve decreased levels of cholinergic receptors, reduced synthesis and release of acetylcholine, and a marked decrease in the number of muscarinic cholinergic neurons, all which may be linked to the age-related memory deficits, a typical change in

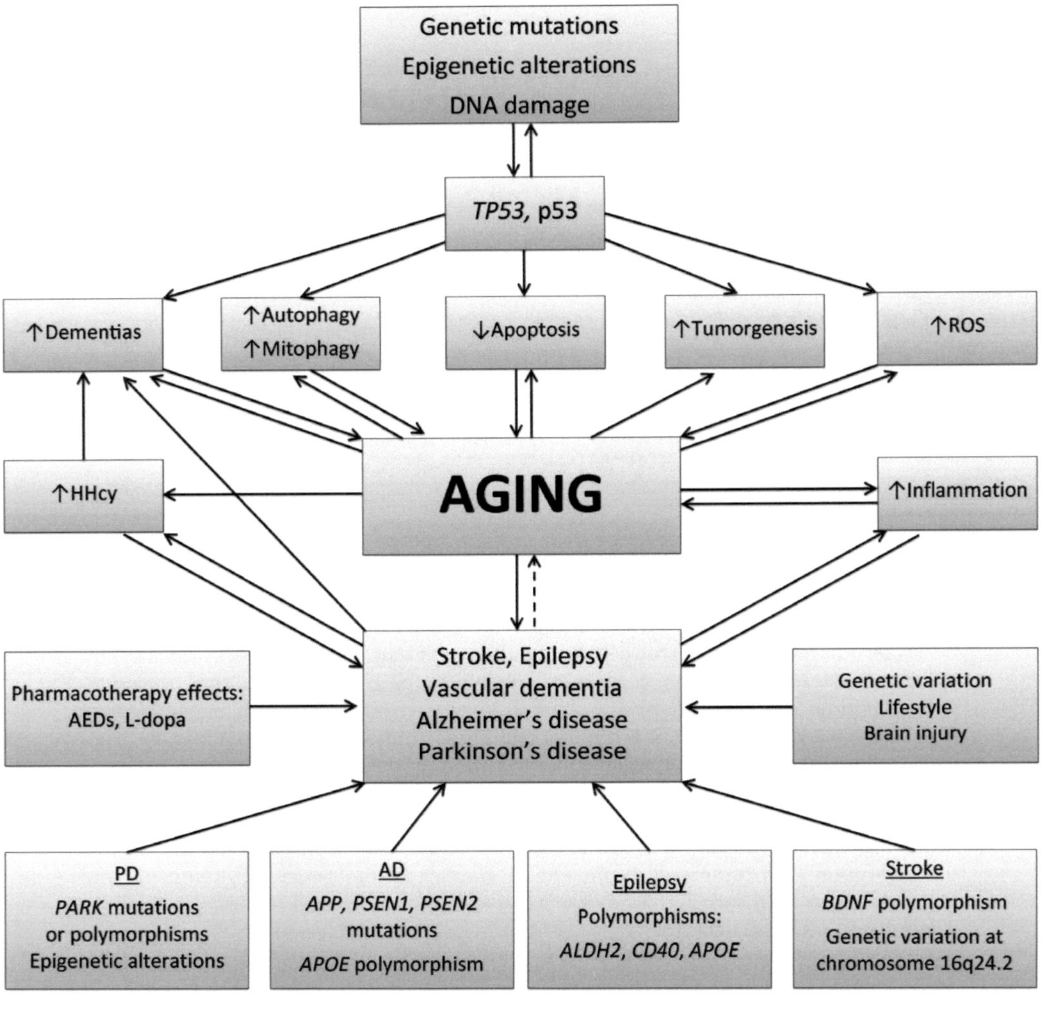

Figure 1. Molecular factors associated with aging and age-related neurological diseases. The pathological changes starting at the molecular level induce oxidative stress and disturb cell cycle that affects cells of the aging organism and lead to systemic deterioration. The genetic variation may give rise to age-related neurological diseases. ROS—reactive oxygen species, HHcy—hyperhomocysteinemia, AEDs—antiepileptic drugs, AD—Alzheimer's disease, and PD—Parkinson's disease.

Alzheimer's disease (AD) patients. Moreover, a decrease in the levels of dopaminergic neurons of up to 40–50% may be observed in the *substantia nigra* and of dopamine in the striatum at the end of the sixth decade of life, which are typical changes seen in patients with Parkinson's disease (PD).

Increased longevity in much of the developed world appears to have lead to higher stroke incidence. Apart from an aging population, there is a significant impact of the growing prevalence of hypertension, diabetes, obesity, and disorders of the cardiovascular system on the increase in the incidence of stroke. The prevalence of these diseases increases with age.

The most common causes of epilepsy in the elderly are vascular changes in the brain (approximately 5%) and degenerative diseases of the central nervous system (CNS) (10–20%). Seizures also occur in patients with AD, demyelinating diseases (multiple sclerosis, or MS), metabolic disorders, as well as in toxic and hormonal disorders, or in individuals with a history of brain injuries or CNS infection.

The mechanisms leading to the development of neurological disorders in the elderly have not been fully elucidated. There are no known mechanisms that regulate cell death in the aging brain. It is not known whether the age of various cells induces the process of apoptosis and other mechanisms of neuronal death, and what factors determine the susceptibility to developing neurological diseases in old age. Understanding the causes of the increased incidence of neurological diseases in the elderly may help in their prevention and improve quality of life in old age (**Figure 1**).

The following review is based on literature search through public databases, such as PubMed and Scopus, with the use of keywords: "aging," "molecular mechanism," "neurological diseases," "stroke," "epilepsy," "vascular dementia," "Alzheimer's disease," "Parkinson's disease," and "brain tumor." Subsequently, the authors selected eligible publications and performed further searches through their references in order to find additional articles. The last search was performed in February 2017.

2. The molecular mechanisms of aging

The molecular mechanisms of aging include genome instability as a consequence of the accumulation of gene mutations, telomere attrition, and epigenetic alterations. Interestingly, instability occurs more frequently in some genome regions than in others. The association and interactions between the above mechanisms lead to the functional decline of aging organisms.

2.1. Aging due to DNA damage

The theory of aging establishes that somatic mutations happen randomly during an organism's lifetime and their accumulation eventually affects key functions such as DNA synthesis, degradation, and repair, consequently causing the "error catastrophe." Genetic damage occurs both in nuclear DNA (nDNA) and mitochondrial DNA (mtDNA) [1, 2]. However, mitochondria have an oxidative environment, due to multiple redox reactions in the electron transport chain, and a less efficient DNA repair system, which results in the accumulation of more damaged mDNA than nDNA [3, 4]. The decreased activity of autophagy and mitophagy may also be responsible for the accumulation of mtDNA mutations and mitochondrial dysfunction during aging [5].

The integrity and stability of DNA may be disrupted both by exogenous factors, such as physical, chemical or biological agents, as well as endogenous factors, including DNA replication errors and reactive oxygen species (ROS) [6]. Most of the damage to DNA occurs during the replication process, and the majority of this damage is corrected by a complex network of DNA repair mechanisms. The mismatch repair (MMR) system provides the fidelity of replication. The checkpoint response is activated by damage that is unrepaired and leads to cell senescence or death, which may also alter tissue and the homeostasis of the body. The loss of key MMR proteins has been observed during aging. The question becomes: is such deterioration a cause or an effect of senescence [7, 8]?

The cell cycle and repair processes are controlled by tumor protein 53 (p53, encoded by *TP53* gene), which is a pivotal regulator of multiple cellular processes, such as reversible and irreversible cell cycle arrest and senescence. The protein is activated by various stress factors to induce apoptosis or autophagic cell death, depending on the cell category [9]. The initiation of cellular aging is designed to prevent proliferation of damaged cells and tumorigenesis. Two main groups of signals activate p53: DNA damage and oncogenic stress. It has been demonstrated that loss of p53 function occurs in senescent cells, as 50% of human neoplasms possesses a mutated copy of the *TP53* gene [10]. Moreover, the mutations in *TP53* were observed also in age-related dementias, such as AD in both humans and its murine model [11, 12] (**Figure 1**).

2.2. The role of telomeres

Telomere attrition is another molecular mechanism responsible for senescence. Telomeres are a structural component of chromosomes localized at the end of each chromatid. They consist of DNA and telomere binding proteins. Telomere DNA is made up of the sequence 5′-TTAGGG-3′ repeated 150–2000 times [13]. The main functions of telomeres are protection against loss of genetic information during replication and prevention of abnormal recombination, chromosome fusion, or chromosomal degradation by exonucleases [14]. During each cell division, the telomere sequence is shortened by a length of 50–200 base pairs (bp) and the structure of telomeres changes. This biological clock is considered to be one of the main mechanisms determining the number of possible cell divisions. Hayflick's observations [15] on somatic cells specified the maximum number of divisions after which cells stop dividing but remain metabolically active. This maximum number is called the Hayflick limit and varies by tissue type and organism. It is known that a reduction in the number of divisions prevents the accumulation of mutations [16].

2.3. Epigenetics of aging

Epigenetic alterations are another molecular mechanism involved in aging and include DNA methylation and histone modifications [17]. The epigenome becomes deregulated with age. Global levels of DNA methylation decrease with age, and changes in the methylation profile may lead to age-associated immune deficiency [18]. The chemical modification of histones includes acetylation, methylation, phosphorylation, ubiquitination, deamination, citrullination, sumoylation, ADP (adenosine diphosphate) ribosylation, and proline isomerization and lead to changes in histone-DNA or histone-histone interactions [19]. Both changes in the DNA methylation pattern and histone modifications can directly alter chromatin packaging, resulting in different parts of the DNA being exposed to transcriptional factors and results in the expression of different genes. Epigenetic studies have demonstrated progressive changes at the transcriptomic level associated with aging. The age range of 49–56 years in humans seems to be critical in transcriptional senescence. Changes in gene expression, either their increase or decrease, are a longitudinal and dynamic process [20] (**Figure 1**).

2.4. Aging of the brain

Furthermore, senescence comprises aging of the cerebral white matter (WM) and gray matter (GM), including progressive neuronal loss, decreased levels of neurotransmitters, increased inflammation, disrupted integrity, lesions, infarction, and microbleeds [21]. Aging affects not only neurons but also glial cells (astrocytes, oligodendrocytes, microglia), vascular cells, and the basal lamina matrix and interferes with their functions such as maintaining metabolic and ion homeostasis in the CNS, regulating the cerebral blood flow, impulse conduction, and phagocytosis [22]. During aging, the reduction of WM volume is almost threefold higher (loss of 28% of neurons) than the reduction of GM volume (10% of neurons). Thus, changes in WM may result in behavioral and cognitive decline in the elderly. Additionally, the ability for WM repair has been found to be decreased in older individuals. Changes in WM are observed in diseases, such as stroke, PD, and AD [21].

Multiple molecular changes take place during aging, and these form a vast network of interactions. This makes it nearly impossible to determine if age-related diseases are caused by a snowball effect of senescence, or if the converse is true: that these diseases are the result of individual variability. It seems that both hypotheses may be true, as aging is an important risk factor for diseases such as stroke, epilepsy, PD, AD, and brain tumors, but not a certain causative factor (**Figure 1**).

3. Neurological diseases associated with aging

3.1. Stroke

According to World Health Organization (WHO), stroke is defined as "rapidly developing clinical signs of focal (or global) disturbance of cerebral function, lasting more than 24 hours or leading to death, with no apparent cause other than that of vascular origin" [23]. There are two main types of stroke, ischemic and hemorrhagic, which have different pathogenesis.

3.1.1. Ischemic and hemorrhagic stroke

In an ischemic stroke, the blood supply to some brain areas is reduced due to narrowing or complete occlusion of arteries, which leads to dysfunction of this part of the brain tissue. The molecular mechanisms involved in the pathomechanism of ischemic stroke include progressive damage of the blood-brain barrier (BBB) due to loss of integrity, degeneration or death of neurons, glial reaction, and infiltration of immune cells. Ischemic stroke represents 85–90% cases of stroke [24, 25]. Age-related changes in WM are thought to increase the risk for stroke, poststroke death [26], and ischemic injury after stroke [27]. One of the molecular features of ischemic stroke in the elderly is excitotoxicity due to changes in protein expression (e.g. increase in GLT-1, a transporter for glutamate) and production of ROS. The generation of ROS leads to the death of oligodendrocytes and to the disruption of axons within WM. In the aged brain, the functional decline of mitochondria and antioxidant systems is associated with greater oxidative stress and worsen the WM injury upon ischemia [21].

Hemorrhagic stroke may be caused by cerebral hemorrhage and subarachnoid hemorrhage as a result of damage to the brain's blood vessels by chronic hypertension, cerebral arteriovenous malformation, intracranial aneurysm, disambiguation, cerebral amyloid angiopathy, or drug-induced bleeding. The molecular basis of such a hemorrhage is represented by cytotoxicity of blood, hypermetabolism, excitotoxicity, oxidative stress, and inflammation [28, 29].

3.1.2. Senescence, civilization diseases, and stroke

The American Heart Association has reported that stroke is the fifth cause of death in the United States [30]. The risk factors of stroke are divided into modifiable (e.g. hypertension and other cardiovascular diseases, migraine, diabetes, dyslipidemia, diet, addictions) and unmodifiable (age, sex, race, genetic factors). Among the unmodifiable risk factors, the most important is age [31]. The risk of stroke increases exponentially with age in both men and women. It is estimated that the incidence of stroke doubles with each decade of life after the age of 55 and affects as many as 5% of people over the age of 65 [32]. It is known that the majority of modifiable risk factors, such as hypertension, atrial fibrillation, hyperhomocysteinemia (HHcy), and inflammatory processes (e.g. periodontal disease, infections, increased hs-CRP), are more common in the elderly. The effect of aging on the cardiovascular system is cumulative [33]. Atrial fibrillation occurs in 5% of individuals aged 70 or above and is a cause of one quarter of stroke incidents in patients at the age of 80. The risk of stroke can be decreased by antithrombotic therapies [34].

The serum total homocysteine (Hcy) concentration is another independent risk factor of ischemic stroke in the elderly, as it correlates with thrombosis. The population attributable risk of stroke incidence in high Hcy levels (>17.4 μmol/L) changes with age and was estimated at 21 and 26% for age 40–59 years (men and women, respectively) and at 35 and 37% for individuals over 60 years of age (men and women, respectively) [35]. HHcy (level of Hcy more than 15.0 μmol/L) promotes the development of atherosclerosis. Clinical studies have shown that HHcy has a toxic impact on both the vascular and nervous systems and may be observed not only in stroke but also in PD, mild cognitive impairment (MCI), and epilepsy [36]. Supplementation of folate and vitamin B_{12} is essential in the treatment of HHcy, but folate alone does not reduce the risk of stroke [37].

Two thirds of the population aged over 65 years suffers from hypertension [31]. Hypertension has been proven to increase fourfold the risk of stroke; as the blood pressure increases, so does the probability of suffering stroke. Fortunately, a blood pressure reduction of about 10/5 mmHg decreases the risk of stroke by about 35% [33]. Hypertension is often linked with obesity, abnormalities in lipid profile, and type 2 diabetes. Together, these comorbidities contribute to atherosclerosis and thromboembolic stroke.

Diabetes has been found to have a greater impact in developing stroke in women than in men. Diabetes is a significant independent contributor of stroke in older women [38, 39]. However, the risk of stroke in diabetic patients can be decreased with proper intervention and treatment. The Systolic Hypertension in the Elderly Program has shown that antihypertensive treatment in individuals with diabetes can reduce the risk of stroke by about 20% [40].

Disturbances in the lipid profile should be regularly reviewed and treated as necessary, as they are another contributor to stroke. Independent studies have shown that high levels of total cholesterol (in the 240–270 mg/dL range) [41–43] and triglycerides [44, 45] as well as a low level of high-density lipoproteins (HDL, up to 35 mg/dL) [43, 46, 47] increase the incidence of ischemic stroke. According to the Heart Protection Study, statin therapy in the elderly group can reduce the risk of a first stroke by 29% [48]. Another side of the coin is obesity, defined as body mass index (BMI) >30 kg/m^2, or abdominal obesity, defined by a waist circumference >102 cm (men) and >88 cm (women) [33]. It is known that abdominal obesity is a stronger predictor of stroke than BMI [49].

Moreover, it has been observed that infection with some pathogens may cause acute stroke within a week; these pathogens are *Chlamydophila pneumoniae, Haemophilus influenzae, Mycoplasma pneumoniae, Helicobacter pylori*, Cytomegalovirus, Epstein-Barr virus, and Herpes simplex virus types I and II. This occurs due to the activation of leukocytes and increased tendency for thrombosis at the site of atherosclerotic plaque. Because of immune deficiencies, the elderly are more susceptible to infections and, therefore, to postinfection complications [33].

It should be mentioned that controlling and regulating the modifiable risk factors is extremely important in stroke prevention. Older people tend to pay more attention to stroke avoidance. Epidemiological studies performed in the USA assumed that, in the last decade, the stroke death rate declined more in subjects after the age of 65 than in the younger population [30].

Stroke is a heterogeneous syndrome, with possible genetic background. Single-gene diseases may cause rare, hereditary disorders for which stroke may be a primary manifestation. Recent studies suggest that common and rare genetic polymorphisms that induce diabetes, hyperlipidemia, or hypertension may activate specific stroke mechanisms causing dangerous angiopathies [50]. For instance, the genetic variation at chromosome 16 (locus q24.2) had been shown to induce small vessel stroke. Traylor et al. using modern GWAS method have found that rare variant rs12445022 in *ZCCHC14* gene may induce small vessels dysfunction, thus greatly increase the risk of stroke [51]. Another interesting genetic factor studied in stroke is a polymorphism in *BDNF* gene (rs6265), which results in amino acid change (Val→Met) in the precursor protein, causing a reduction in brain-derived neurotrophic factor (BDNF) activity, which plays a role in rehabilitation after stroke. The studies show that concentrations of BDNF were decreased in acute ischemic-stroke patients compared to controls. BDNF signaling is dependent on the genetic variation which could affect an individual's response to recovery after stroke. The rs6265 polymorphism may also affect the risk of ischemic stroke, post-stroke outcomes and the efficacy of the various forms of rehabilitation [52] (**Figure 1**).

3.2. Epilepsy

Epilepsy is one of the most common neurological diseases, with approximately 50 million sufferers worldwide. Epilepsy is a collection of somatic, vegetative, and/or mental symptoms, which may be the result of morphological or metabolic changes in the brain. Although the disease has a chronic character and had long been thought to be connected with events in infancy or childhood, epidemiological studies have revealed that there is pronounced incidence of epilepsy in people over 65 years of age [53, 54]. To date, many various causative factors have been associated with epilepsy. However, the etiology of the disease remains unknown in 65–75% of patients [55].

Epilepsy that develops after the age of 60 is symptomatic in the vast majority, although generalized epilepsy may also rarely manifest in the elderly [56]. Epileptic seizures are often underdiagnosed in that age group. The symptoms are usually recognized as memory disorders or mental changes of uncertain origin [57]. Risk factors for epilepsy and seizure etiology vary with age. The most common mechanism of pathogenesis of new-onset epilepsy and seizures in the elderly may be associated with cerebrovascular diseases (CVDs), neuron degenerative disorders, intracerebral tumors, and traumatic head injury [58, 59].

3.2.1. Epilepsy and cerebrovascular diseases

CVDs account for 30–50% of all identified causes of epilepsy in the elderly [60, 61]. Epilepsy attacks may be affected by a stroke and may occur immediately after an ischemic event or be delayed. Seizures may also be the first clinical manifestation of brain ischemia or hemorrhage, increasing the risk to develop epilepsy within the first year after the vascular episode by 20 times. The study of Alberti et al. [62] showed that hemorrhagic transformation of an ischemic stroke is a predictive factor for epilepsy and may also be related to the disruption of the BBB [63]. Numerous genetic factors may be engaged in epileptogenesis. According to Yang et al. [64], mitochondrial aldehyde dehydrogenase 2 (ALDH2, encoded by the *ALDH2* gene) has a protective effect in CVDs. Nevertheless, allele A of the rs671 polymorphism in the *ALDH2* gene was shown to be connected with post-stroke epilepsy due to decreased activity of ALDH2 leading to accumulation of the potential ALDH2 substrate—4-hydroxynonenal (4-HNE), considered to be a specific marker of oxidative stress and involved in myocardial and cerebral ischemia. Zhang et al. [65] suggest that the T allele of the -1C/T polymorphism in the *CD40* gene may be associated with susceptibility to poststroke epilepsy (**Figure 1**). The proposed mechanism includes raised plasma concentrations of sCD40L, which is involved in the inflammatory response. Moreover, poststroke epileptogenesis was shown to be associated with lifestyle factors (alcohol use), acute metabolic disturbances (hyperglycemia), non-CNS comorbidities (type 1 or 2 diabetes, hypertension, coronary heart disease or myocardial infarction, as well as peripheral infections), CNS diseases (early seizures, depression or use of antidepressants, dementia), and pharmacotherapy (statins) [66].

3.2.2. Epilepsy due to head trauma

Another causative factor of epilepsy in the elderly may be head trauma. Due to an increased likelihood of imbalance, older people are more prone to falls causing head injuries. Acute events, such as skull fractures, subdural hematoma, brain contusion, accidental injury, concussion, or loss of consciousness, were shown to be associated with increased risk of posttraumatic epilepsy [67]. Moreover, various genetic factors were shown to be associated with head injury as a risk factor for late posttraumatic seizures. Diaz-Arrastia et al. [68] showed that carriers of the pathogenic *APOE* E4 allele were more likely to develop epilepsy after suffering acute head trauma (**Figure 1**).

3.2.3. Epilepsy due to brain tumor

Epileptic seizures are common symptoms of brain tumors (BTs) in 20–40% of patients. The study of de Assis et al. [69] demonstrates that BTs related to epilepsy include primary CNS lymphoma, meningioma, anaplastic ependymoma, and anaplastic astrocytoma. The highest incidence of epilepsy occurs in low-grade tumors like primary astrocytoma, oligodendroglioma, mixed astrocytoma WHO grade I and II, as well as meningiomas. It seems that the incidence of seizures is inversely correlated to the grade of the malignancy. Age is a risk factor for increased mortality in those BT patients who develop seizures. Epilepsy attacks also appear in 67% of patients with melanocytic brain metastases, in 48% patients with lung cancer metastases, in 33% patients with breast cancer, and in 55% of patients in whom the primary cancer type was unknown. Unfortunately, BT-related epilepsy is characterized by pharmacological resistance [69, 70].

3.2.4. Biochemical factors in epilepsy

Hcy seems to have additional and interesting significance for the development of epilepsy. As stated earlier, HHcy has demonstrated an association with several disorders, including epilepsy [71]. High Hcy concentration has been shown to be related to numerous factors, including lifestyle (smoking, high consumption of alcohol, caffeine), age (due to the weakening of the excretory function of the kidneys, malabsorption of vitamin B_{12} in the stomach, hormonal disorders, e.g. in women during and after menopause), comorbid diseases, pharmacotherapy (e.g. antidiabetic drugs or fibrates), or unbalanced diet (deficiency of vitamin B_{12} or folic acid) [72–75]. Moreover, Schwaninger et al. [76] demonstrated that prolonged treatment with antiepileptic drugs (AEDs) may increase the plasma concentration of Hcy. On the other hand, the authors were not able to conclude whether the HHcy in epilepsy patients was a sole effect of pharmacotherapy or a causative factor of the disease.

Seizures may also occur in metabolic disorders, because of multiple comorbidities and polypharmacy. There should be a high index of suspicion for electrolyte imbalance, especially hyponatremia and hypoglycemia, in this group of patients. Other metabolic disorders, such as hyperglycemia and uremic or hepatic encephalopathy, are less specific to this age group [77]. The role of alcohol appears to be less important in the elderly than in young adults, but should not be neglected [78], as it may intensify the number of calcium channels and promote seizure activity by increasing the concentration of neurotransmitters [79].

3.2.5. Epilepsy in degenerative diseases

AD is a significant risk factor of epilepsy in the elderly. Imfeld et al. [80] suggested that patients with a longer history of AD (≥3 years) may have a higher risk of developing seizures or epilepsy than those with a shorter duration of disease. Similar results were presented by Amatniek et al. [81], who observed that the incidence of seizures increased as the disease progressed; the cumulative incidence over 7 years was 8%. The risk of seizure onset is higher in AD patients with hyperlipidemia and severe dementia [82]. The epileptogenetic mechanism has not yet been elucidated in patients with neurodegeneration. It might be associated with β-amyloid (Aβ) deposition, neuronal loss and gliosis, and antidementia drugs [83, 84]. High levels of Aβ are considered a cause of AD, but they are also related to synaptic activity. Aβ serves as a potent regulator of synaptic transmission, causing presynaptic facilitation at relatively low Aβ concentrations and postsynaptic depression with higher Aβ levels. The modulation of synaptic transmission has an important effect on producing epileptiform activity [85].

Another degenerative disorder which may potentially induce seizures is MS, a chronic disease of the CNS. MS usually occurs in young adults (aged 20 to 40 years). However, 1.1–12% of MS patients experience the first symptoms of the disease after the age of 50 [86]. The prevalence of seizures among MS patients was shown to be higher than the general population, which may indicate the relationship between seizures and MS [87]. One possible explanation is that MS lesions act as epileptogenic sites [88]. Generally, a small fraction (2.5%) of MS patients develop seizures [89]. The study of epilepsy in the elderly among MS patients is inconclusive, but clinicians should be aware of the risk of epilepsy in people with MS [88].

3.3. Aging and dementia

Dementia—as a form of cognitive decline—is strongly associated with old age. Almost 10% of those older than 65 years suffer from some kind of memory impairment. The most common causes of dementia include AD and vascular dementia (VaD). The prevalence of dementia increases with age, affecting nearly 50% of the population over 85 years of age. Dementia is a progressive disorder, finally leading to severe disability and complete dependence of sufferers on caregivers [90].

3.3.1. Vascular dementia

VaD was initially understood to be an advanced effect of repetitive brain lesions [91]. The development of brain imaging techniques revealed that silent ischemic lesions appeared to be quite common and later became known as a significant cause of dementia [92, 93]. Epidemiological studies have shown that vascular dysfunction causes 10–20% dementia cases [94, 95]. The frequency of VaD in the general population varies from 1.2 to 4.2% of individuals over 65 years, depending on the methodological approach [94, 96]. The prevalence of VaD is strongly connected with age. A Canadian study described that frequency of vascular cognitive impairment increased from 2.0% in those aged 65 to 74 years to 13.7% in those over 85 years of age [97]. A meta-analysis from 1998, synthesizing the results of 23 studies from around the world, confirmed the trend of increasing incidence of VaD in senescence [98]. Increasing longevity in many populations has also increased the importance and burden of vascular-related memory deficits. A long-term survey demonstrated that the incidence of post-stroke dementia between 1984 and 2001 had doubled [99].

Several studies have analyzed the risk factors, other than age, of CNS vascular lesions. They identified hypertension, heart disease, diabetes with insulin resistance, and dyslipidemia to be related to an increased risk to develop VaD. It is important to note that the results obtained by different authors occasionally contradict each other [100–109]. The cluster of cardiovascular risk factors, also called "metabolic syndrome," that include dyslipidemia, obesity, hypertension, and insulin resistance, has also been shown to be associated with VaD [110, 111]. Additionally, patients with fully symptomatic metabolic syndrome obtained lesser scores in neuropsychological testing [112]. Moreover, HHcy, previously associated with vascular diseases and stroke, was shown to be associated with VaD [113].

Many studies have also demonstrated that a symptomatic stroke incident, occurring mostly in the elderly, may inflict memory deficits in 6 to 32% of patients, depending on the follow-up period (3 months—20 years) [114–128]. MCI preceding stroke increases the probability of post-stroke dementia [129, 130], and memory decline seemed to progress more rapidly with later stroke episodes [131]. Similarly, recurrent stroke was associated with greater cognitive impairment when compared with patients with a single vascular incident [122] (**Figure 1**).

3.3.2. Alzheimer's disease

AD is the most common form of dementia in older adults [132]. AD is a progressive incurable neurodegenerative disease where aging is the primary risk factor. AD may be divided into two main clinical subtypes: familial AD (FAD) characterized by early onset (before 65 years of age) and, frequently, the presence of mutations in the *APP*, *PSEN1*, and *PSEN2* genes. This genetic triad is responsible for nearly half of the FAD cases seen [133]. However, mutations in these genes occur very rarely in the human population. Subsequently, the majority (90%) of AD cases are sporadic (SAD) and manifest mostly in patients over 65 years of age. The multifactorial character of the disease makes it extremely difficult to determine a causative factor for SAD [134]. To date, nearly 700 genes have been associated with AD, although the most investigated risk factor for SAD remains the E4 allele of the *APOE* gene [90, 135, 136].

The diagnosis of probable AD is based on clinical criteria [137], however, the disease may be diagnosed with certainty only after death, by histopathologic study of the brain, revealing characteristic lesions: Aβ plaques and neurofibrillary tangles (NFTs) formed by hyperphosphorylated protein tau. Aβ is formed via pathologic cleavage of (amyloid precursor protein (APP), encoded by the *APP* gene) by β- and γ-secretases (encoded by the *BACE* and *PSEN* genes, respectively). The appearance of Aβ plaques and NFTs seems to be one of the causes for neurodegeneration: the morphological and functional loss of neurons and synapses, as well as excessive neuroinflammatory processes occurring in AD brains. Martin et al. [138] showed that aging and Aβ pathology may activate similar receptors on microglia and monocyte-derived macrophages. Moreover, carriers of the *APOE* E4 allele and rare variants in other genes, such as *HLA-DRB5/DRB1*, *INPP5D*, *MEF2C*, *CR1*, *CLU*, and *TREM2*, may exhibit an even stronger activation of microglia than noncarriers [139]. This explains why older patients with unfavorable genetic variants are more prone to excessive neuroinflammatory responses leading to neuronal loss and dementia.

The neurons mostly affected by AD are cells expressing acetylcholine (ACh) receptors, also called "cholinergic neurons" (AChN). Loss and degeneration of this type of cells is another hallmark of dementia and occurs gradually with age and the course of the disease [140]. The age-related degeneration of AChN leads to decreasing levels of ACh in the brain. ACh has been proven to be the neurotransmitter that is most reduced in the majority of AD patients [141]. It seems that genetic factors, such as the presence of the pathogenic *APOE* E4 allele, may also significantly influence the production and release of ACh. The study on transgenic mice expressing human *APOE* indicated that age-related decrease in ACh levels released by the hippocampus was more prominent in mice with human *APOE* E4/E4 than in mice with *APOE* E3/E3 variants [142] (**Figure 1**).

The main cholinergic structure of the brain is the basal forebrain (BF), the underlying neurodegeneration of which may be observed in advanced aging as well as in the early phase of AD and other dementias [143]. BF degeneration occurs due to a decrease in cholinergic neurotransmission and a reduction in the amount of ACh in synaptic clefts, followed by a loss of cholinergic receptors, finally resulting in AChN death. This process, according to the "cholinergic deficit hypothesis," results in behavioral and cognitive impairment, especially learning difficulties, which advance rapidly with age [144].

It is worth noting that in AD, similarly to VaD and stroke, the concentration of Hcy may be increased and so may inflict damage to the vasculature, thereby leading to decreased blood flow and inefficient nutrient delivery to neurons. Subsequently, the starving cells become more prone to ROS and apoptosis. HHcy is also associated with a decrease of the glutathione pool, the deficiency of which results in the deterioration of protection mechanisms from free radicals, further contributing to neuronal loss and neurodegeneration [145].

3.4. Parkinson's disease and aging

PD is an age-related neurodegenerative disease characterized by resting tremor, rigidity, and bradykinesia. The number of PD patients increases over the years due to population aging. The exact pathomechanism of PD remains unclear, but it is known that the degeneration process starts many years before the occurrence of clinical symptoms. The hallmark of PD is dopaminergic (DA) neuron death in the substantia nigra (SN), which is a result of Lewy body (LB) formation due to impairment of the ubiquitin-proteasome system and disturbances in the proteins alpha-synuclein (ASN) and Parkin [146, 147]. Molecular characteristic of PD include increased ROS production due to mitochondrial dysfunction and accompanied by decreased mitophagy [148], neuroinflammation and loss of neurotrophic factors [149, 150], exposure to (1-methyl-4-phenyl-1, 2,3,6-tetrahydropyridine (MPTP)) or paraquat [151], exposure to trichloroethylene or polychlorinated biphenyls [152], iron (the level of which increase in the SN with age), copper, manganese [153, 154], or mutations in *PARK* genes [155]. Mitochondrial dysfunction is associated with aggregation of ASN, apoptosis, accumulation of damaged mitochondria, and changes in the activity of complex 1 [156]. A decline in mitochondrial function as well as inflammation and changes in DA metabolism are linked with the aging process.

Advancing age is the most important risk factor of developing PD. PD affects about 1% of the population over the age of 60 and 5% over the age of 85 [157]. It has been since 1987 that the loss of DA neurons progresses with aging, but the rate of the physiological process is slower than that seen in PD [158]. Moreover, LB may be present in elderly individuals without PD [159]. The aging brain is also more prone to stressor stimuli and generation of ROS, which results in the injury and eventual death of SN neurons. On the other hand, a decreased level or even loss of ROS scavengers, e.g. neuromelanin, in the PD brain may be a cause of DA neuron damage rather than an effect of this damage [157].

Many epigenetic mechanisms, such as changes in DNA methylation profile and histone modification, play an important role in aging and contribute to PD. The epigenetic clock can be characterized just by measuring the DNA methylation pattern. Interestingly, PD patients represent an increased acceleration in aging when compared to controls of the same age [160]. Hypomethylation of *SNCA*, the gene encoding ASN, leads to an increased expression of ASN and has been observed in the SN of PD patients [161]. ASN can also influence histone acetylation (a feature of transcriptionally active genes) and enhance ASN fibrillation [162].

During normal aging, the functional decline of the BBB can cause neuroinflammation and the development of neurodegenerative diseases [163]. Disturbances in BBB permeability observed in the senescence process may be involved in the genesis of WM lesions, which may also affect the efficacy of treatment. In the course of aggregation of ASN in PD, elevated ROS production and increased levels of proinflammatory cytokines or toxic agents may intensify disruptions of the BBB [164].

HHcy observed in PD may be involved in the disease pathogenesis; however, the exact mechanism of interaction remains unrecognized. Both HHcy and age are risk factors for developing dementia in PD patients [165]. Treatment with L-dopa may be responsible for HHcy in individuals with PD [166]. In those patients, Hcy is formed in the methylation of L-dopa via catechol-O-methyltransferase (COMT) [167]. Other side effects of L-dopa at the molecular level include increased oxidative stress, as well as altered concentrations of catecholamines and apoptotic proteins [147]. Damage of DA neurons due to oxidative stress may be enhanced by elevated Hcy (**Figure 1**). A study performed on mice has shown that elevated Hcy increases the sensitivity to MPTP and developing PD-like dysfunction [168].

3.5. Brain tumors in the elderly

Another type of CNS disease, manifesting particularly in the elderly, are brain tumors, classified according to WHO criteria to four grades, with grade IV considered most malignant [169]. In adults, the most prevalent type of primary brain tumor is malignant glioma (MGs), with the highest incidence between 40 and 65 years of age. The majority of MGs are sporadic, with ionizing radiation as the only known risk factor. The most common type of glioma is glioblastoma multiforme (GBM), qualified as a WHO grade IV astrocytic tumor, and constituting about half of all MGs with the highest incidence in the elderly, between 70 and 90 years of age [170–172]. Old age is a negative prognostic factor in GBM [173]. One of the most significant characteristics of GBM is an increasing prevalence with age; thus, due to an increasing median length of life, the number of patients is expected to grow in the coming decades. Other types of brain tumors common in the elderly are primary CNS lymphomas (PCNSLs) and meningiomas [174].

GBM comprise a rather heterogenic group of neoplasms, with two major types: primary glioblastomas (85–90%) and secondary GBMs that arise from low-grade astrocytomas (10–15%) [175]. Although both types are indistinguishable under the microscope, they appear to differ genetically. Genetically, primary GBMs exhibit by amplification and mutation of the *EGFR* gene, a lack of heterozygosity on chromosome 10q, inactivation of the *PTEN* homolog gene, and only rare occurrence of mutations in the *IDH* and *TP53* genes. Conversely, the genetics of secondary GBM are characterized by mutations in the *IDH* and/or *TP53* genes, as well as platelet-derived growth factor receptor activation [176]. A gene expression-based GBM classification was established by The Cancer Genome Atlas (TCGA) Research Network in 2010. The authors distinguished four subtypes of GBM. Characteristics that differentiate the subtypes at most were indicated as follows: proneural GBM has alterations of the *PDGFRA* gene and point mutations of *IDH1*, classical GBM has *EGFR* aberrations, and mesenchymal demonstrates GBM aberrations in *NF1*. The fourth subtype, neural GBM, is characterized by the expression of neuron markers such as *NEFL, GABRA1, SYT1,* and *SLC12A5*. Each subtype of GBM differs in its sensitivity to radiotherapy and chemotherapy, thus determining the genetic type of a surgically removed or biopsied lesion could protect patients against unnecessary ineffective therapy [177].

Unfortunately, GBMs are mostly incurable in the elderly, with most of these patients surviving less than 6 months [171]. Diagnosis of primary brain tumors in old age can be further complicated and delayed due to nonspecific symptoms that can be masked by physical and cognitive changes observed in the normal aging process [178]. Moreover, elderly patients are an underrepresented group in many clinical trials [179]. The literature data indicate that, at the close of the twentieth century, the chances of receiving a treatment, be that surgery and/or radiotherapy, were decreasing as the patient got older. Treatment mostly took place for 82% of patients younger than 65 years of age, whereas only 47% of people older than 65 years and merely 25% of patients older than 75 were subjected to any kind of therapy. Additionally, patients treated with radiotherapy and/or surgery had a significantly lower survival rate as they crossed the age border of 60 years [180].

Although pathological processes differ depending on the glioma subtype, there is a common core of molecular events. Growth factor receptor tyrosine kinases cause downstream signaling by activation of extracellular signal-regulated kinases (ERK) or protein kinase B (Akt) pathways. Lack of p53 activation is followed by the loss of the ability to activate DNA repair processes and cell death by apoptosis. An additional adverse characteristic occurring in GBM is that the cells provoke the secretion of vascular endothelial growth factor (VEGF), which is responsible for angiogenesis. The secretion of VEGF by GBM results in vascularization of the tumor, elevation of capillary permeability of the BBB, and creation of extracellular edema [181]. Finally, due to vasculature growth, there is progression of tumor invasion [182].

Although these brain tumors are very invasive, it is important to note that, depending on the tumor subtype, they may be effectively treated in elderly patients by maximally safe surgical resection, radiotherapy, and/or chemotherapy with Temozolomide, a drug which is especially preferable as first-line treatment in patients with the *MGMT* promoter [179, 183]. In addition to radiotherapy and/or Temozolomide, Bevacizumab (BV, Avastin®) is being studied for the treatment of brain tumors. BV is a humanized IgG1 monoclonal antibody targeting VEGF with high affinity and inactivating the growth factor. Thus, BV promotes tumor regression and helps to decrease the risk of cerebral edema [184]. Interestingly, it has been demonstrated that, although old age is a negative prognostic factor, BV was more effective in older patients (≥55 years of age); those treated with BV remained in better health longer and used lower doses of steroids. These findings were in line with the study published by Nghiemphu et al. [185], who demonstrated that expression of VEGF was 1.4-fold higher in older patients than in younger subjects, and so inhibition of VEGF could give a more positive outcome in these patients.

The increased incidence of brain tumors in the elderly may also be due to decreased efficiency of repair mechanisms. Inactivation of genes involved in DNA repair, such as the above-mentioned *TP53* and *MGMT*, may advance with age. This may lead to increased accumulation of DNA damage, in turn resulting in further activation of proto-oncogenes and silencing of tumor suppressor genes. Such changes, inflicted either by mutation or epigenetic changes, may cause additional destabilization of cellular repair mechanisms, increasing the susceptibility to ROS and spontaneous mutagenesis, and triggering the positive feedback loop of neoplasia [186] (**Figure 1**).

4. Summary

The molecular mechanism of aging includes genome-wide changes such as genomic instability due to accumulation of mutations, telomere attrition, and epigenetic alterations. These changes collect over the years during the life of the organism, leading gradually to morphological and functional deterioration. The brain seems to be particularly vulnerable, as neurons generally do not divide and their pool decreases with the passage of time. Structural changes in the senescent brain affect mostly the cerebral WM and GM; these effects include progressive neuronal loss, decreased levels of neurotransmitters, increased inflammatory processes, and disrupted integrity of vessels and the BBB followed by infarction and microbleeds. These changes may lead to degenerative diseases, such as PD and dementias.

The frequently observed malnutrition and malabsorption syndrome in the elderly may cause decreased concentrations of the vitamins necessary for Hcy metabolism. This in turn results in increased injury to the cerebral vasculature, leading to degeneration and strokes. Consequently, progressive age-related vascular damage of the brain develops, additionally connected to an increased prevalence of epilepsy in the elderly.

An increased incidence of brain tumors may also be observed in old age, probably as an effect of the diminished efficiency of repair mechanisms. The inactivation of genes involved in DNA repair has been shown to advance with age. Such alterations, inflicted either by epigenetic changes or mutation, may cause further destabilization of immunologic systems and cellular repair mechanisms, thus increasing the susceptibility to ROS and spontaneous mutagenesis and resulting in uncontrolled cellular growth and age-related neoplasia (**Figure 2**).

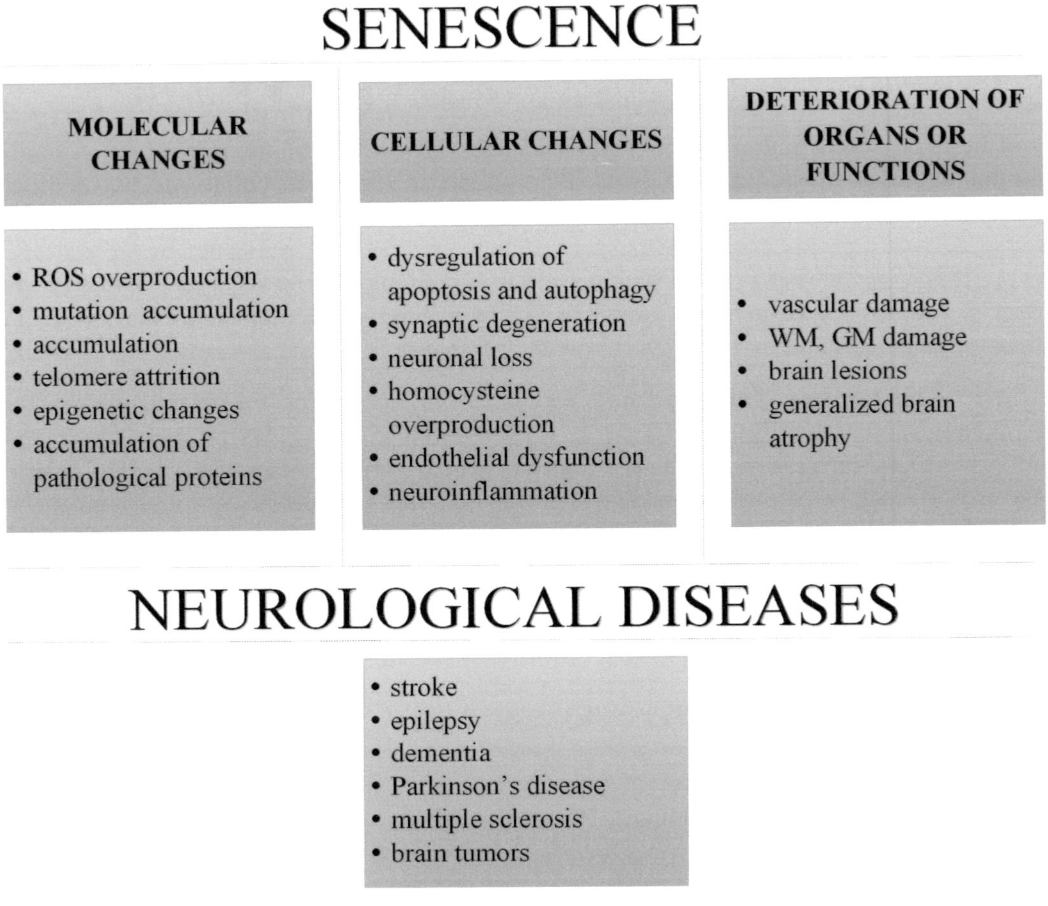

Figure 2. Changes during the senescence process may be associated with neurological diseases. The pathological changes starting at the molecular level affect cells of the aging organism and lead to systemic deterioration, giving rise to age-related neurological diseases. ROS—reactive oxygen species, WM—white matter of the brain, and GM—gray matter of the brain.

In summary, the senescence mechanisms start at a molecular level and gradually lead to morphological disintegration and functional loss of brain cells. Finally, they lead to the deterioration of the CNS and an increased risk of developing neurological diseases.

Acknowledgements

This work was supported by the Poznan University of Medical Sciences grant no. 502-01-11111-45-07-467.

Author details

Marta Kowalska[1], Michal Owecki[1,2], Michal Prendecki[1], Katarzyna Wize[1], Joanna Nowakowska[1], Wojciech Kozubski[3], Margarita Lianeri[1] and Jolanta Dorszewska[1]*

*Address all correspondence to: dorszewskaj@yahoo.com

1 Laboratory of Neurobiology, Department of Neurology, Poznan University of Medical Sciences, Poznan, Poland

2 Chair and Department of History of Medical Sciences, Poznan University of Medical Sciences, Poznan, Poland

3 Chair and Department of Neurology, Poznan University of Medical Sciences, Poznan, Poland

References

[1] Orgel LE. The maintenance of the accuracy of protein synthesis and its relevance to ageing. Proceedings of the National Academy of Sciences USA. 1963;**49**:517-521

[2] Kirkwood TB. Evolution of ageing. Nature. 1977;**270**:301-304

[3] Blasiak J, Glowacki S, Kauppinen A, Kaarniranta K. Mitochondrial and nuclear DNA damage and repair in age-related macular degeneration. International Journal of Molecular Sciences. 2013;**14**:2996-3010. DOI: 10.3390/ijms14022996

[4] Alexeyev M, Shokolenko I, Wilson G, LeDoux S. The maintenance of mitochondrial DNA integrity- critical analysis and update. Cold Spring Harbor Perspectives in Biology. 2013;**5**:a012641. DOI: 10.1101/cshperspect.a012641

[5] Gaziev AI, Abdullaev S, Podlutsky A. Mitochondrial function and mitochondrial DNA maintenance with advancing age. Biogerontology. 2014;**15**:417-438. DOI: 10.1007/s10522-014-9515-2

[6] Hoeijmakers JH. DNA damage, aging, and cancer. New England Journal of Medicine. 2009;**361**:1475-1485. DOI: 10.1056/NEJMra0804615

[7] Hsieh P, Yamane K. DNA mismatch repair: Molecular mechanism, cancer, and ageing. Mechanisms of Ageing and Development. 2008;**129**:391-407. DOI: 10.1016/j.mad.2008.02.012

[8] Ruzankina Y, Asare A, Brown EJ. Replicative stress, stem cells and aging. Mechanisms of Ageing and Development. 2008;**129**:460-466. DOI: 10.1016/j.mad.2008.03.009

[9] Garcia-Cao I, Garcia-Cao M, Martin-Caballero J, Criado LM, Klatt P, Flores JM, Weill JC, Blasco MA, Serrano M (2002) 'Super p53' mice exhibit enhanced DNA damage response, are tumor resistant and age normally. The EMBO Journal. 2002;**21**:6225-6235

[10] Bougeard G., Brugieres L, Chompret A, Gesta P, Charbonnier F, Valent A, Martin C, Raux G, Feunteun J, Bressac-de Paillerets B, Frébourg T. Screening for TP53 rearrangements in families with the Li-Fraumeni syndrome reveals a complete deletion of the TP53 gene. Oncogene. 2003;**22**:840-846

[11] Dorszewska J, Oczkowska A, Suwalska M, Rozycka A, Florczak-Wyspianska J, Dezor M, Lianeri M, Jagodzinski PP, Kowalczyk MJ, Prendecki M, Kozubski W. Mutations in the exon 7 of Trp53 gene and the level of p53 protein in double transgenic mouse model of Alzheimer's disease. Folia Neuropathologica. 2014;**52**:30-40

[12] Dorszewska, J, Różycka A, Oczkowska A, Florczak-Wyspiańska J, Prendecki M, Dezor M, Postrach I, Jagodzinski P, Kozubski W. Mutations of TP53 gene and oxidative stress in Alzheimer's disease patients. Advances in Alzheimer's Disease. 2014;**3**:24-32. DOI: 10.4236/aad.2014.31004

[13] Lu W, Zhang Y, Liu D, Songyang Z, Wan M. Telomeres-structure, function, and regulation. Experimental Cell Research. 2013;**319**:133-141. DOI: 10.1016/j.yexcr.2012.09.005

[14] Martínez P, Blasco MA. Telomeric and extra-telomeric roles for telomerase and the telomere-binding proteins. Nature Reviews Cancer. 2011;**11**:161-176. DOI: 10.1038/nrc3025

[15] Hayflick L. The limited in vitro lifetime of human diploid cell strains. Experimental Cell Research. 1965;**37**:614-636

[16] Chin L, Artandi SE, Shen Q et al. p53 deficiency rescues the adverse effects of telomere loss and cooperates with telomere dysfunction to accelerate carcinogenesis. Cell. 1999;**97**:527-538. DOI: 10.1016/S0092-8674(00)80762-X

[17] Berger SL, Kouzarides T, Shiekhattar R, Shilatifard A. An operational definition of epigenetics. Genes and Development. 2009;**23**:781-783. DOI: 10.1101/gad.1787609

[18] Marttila S, Kananen L, Häyrynen S, Jylhävä J, Nevalainen T, Hervonen A, Jylhä M, Nykter M, Hurme M. Ageing-associated changes in the human DNA methylome: Genomic locations and effects on gene expression. BMC Genomics. 2015;**16**:179. DOI: 10.1186/s12864-015-1381-z

[19] Kouzarides T. Chromatin modifications and their function. Cell. 2007;**128**:693-705. DOI: 10.1016/j.cell.2007.02.005

[20] Irizar H, Goñi J, Alzualde A, Castillo-Triviño T, Olascoaga J, Lopez de Munain A, Otaegui D. Age gene expression and coexpression progressive signatures in peripheral blood leukocytes. Experimental Gerontology. 2015;**72**:50-56. DOI: 10.1016/j.exger.2015.09.003

[21] Liu H, Yang Y, Xia Y, Zhu W, Leak RK, Wei Z, Wang J, Hu X. Aging of cerebral white matter. Ageing Research Reviews. 2017;**34**:64-76. DOI: 10.1016/j.arr.2016.11.006

[22] Cai W, Zhang K, Li P, Zhu L, Xu J, Yang B, Hu X, Lu Z, Chen J. Dysfunction of the neurovascular unit in ischemic stroke and neurodegenerative diseases: An aging effect. Ageing Research Reviews. 2017;**34**:77-87. DOI: 10.1016/j.arr.2016.09.006

[23] Aho K, Harmsen P, Hatano S, Marquardsen J, Smirnov VE, Strasser T. Cerebrovascular disease in the community: Results of a WHO collaborative study. Bull World Health Organ. 1980;**58**:113-130

[24] Rothwell PM, Coull AJ, Giles MF, Howard SC, Silver LE, Bull LM, Gutnikov SA, Edwards P, Mant D, Sackley CM, Farmer A, Sandercock PA, Dennis MS, Warlow CP, Bamford JM, Anslow P. Change in stroke incidence, mortality, case-fatality, severity, and risk factors in Oxfordshire, UK from 1981 to 2004 (Oxford Vascular Study). Lancet. 2004;**363**:1925-1933. DOI: 10.1016/S0140-6736(04)16405-2

[25] Sohrabji F. Bake S, Lewis DK. Age-related changes in brain support cells: Implications for stroke severity. Neurochemistry International. 2004;**63**:291-301. DOI: 10.1016/j.neuint.2013.06.013

[26] Oksala NK, Oksala A, Pohjasvaara T, Vataja R, Kaste M, Karhunen PJ, Erkinjuntti T. Age related white matter changes predict stroke death in long-term follow-up. Journal of Neurology, Neurosurgery and Psychiatry. 2009;**80**:762-766

[27] Rosenzweig S, Carmichael ST. Age-dependent exacerbation of white matter stroke outcomes: A role for oxidative damage and inflammatory mediators. Stroke. 2013;**44**:2579-2586. DOI: 10.1161/STROKEAHA.113.001796

[28] Smith SD, Eskey CJ. Hemorrhagic stroke. Radiologic Clinics of North America. 2011;**49**:27-45. DOI: 10.1016/j.rcl.2010.07.011

[29] Aronowski J, Zhao X. Molecular pathophysiology of cerebral hemorrhage: Secondary brain injury. Stroke. 2011;**42**:1781-1786. DOI: 10.1161/STROKEAHA.110.596718

[30] Mozaffarian D, Benjamin EJ, Go AS, Arnett DK, Blaha MJ, Cushman M, Das SR, de Ferranti S, Després JP, Fullerton HJ, Howard VJ, Huffman MD, Isasi CR, Jiménez MC, Judd SE, Kissela BM, Lichtman JH, Lisabeth LD, Liu S, Mackey RH, Magid DJ, McGuire DK, Mohler ER 3rd, Moy CS, Muntner P, Mussolino ME, Nasir K, Neumar RW, Nichol G, Palaniappan L, Pandey DK, Reeves MJ, Rodriguez CJ, Rosamond W, Sorlie PD, Stein J, Towfighi A, Turan TN, Virani SS, Woo D, Yeh RW, Turner MB. American Heart Association Statistics Committee. Stroke Statistics Subcommittee. Executive Summary: Heart Disease and Stroke Statistics-2016 Update: A report from the American Heart Association. Heart Association. Circulation. 2016;**133**:447-454. DOI: 10.1161/CIR.0000000000000366

[31] Strepikowska A, Buciński A. Cerebral stroke—risk factors and prophylaxis. Postępy farmakoterapii. 2009;**65**:46-50. In Polish

[32] Hirtz D, Thurman DJ, Gwinn-Hardy K, Mohamed M, Chaudhuri AR, Zalutsky R. How common are the 'common' neurologic disorders? Neurology. 2007;**68**:326-337. DOI: 10.1212/01.wnl.0000252807.38124.a3

[33] Goldstein LB, Adams R, Alberts MJ, Appel LJ, Brass LM, Bushnell CD, Culebras A, DeGraba TJ, Gorelick PB, Guyton JR, Hart RG, Howard G, Kelly-Hayes M, Nixon JV, Sacco RL. American Heart Association; American Stroke Association Stroke Council.

Primary prevention of ischemic stroke: A guideline from the American Heart Association/ American Stroke Association Stroke Council: Cosponsored by the Atherosclerotic Peripheral Vascular Disease Interdisciplinary Working Group; Cardiovascular Nursing Council; Clinical Cardiology Council; Nutrition, Physical Activity, and Metabolism Council; and the Quality of Care and Outcomes Research Interdisciplinary Working Group. Circulation. 2006;**113**:e873-e923. DOI: 10.1161/01.STR.0000223048.70103.F1

[34] Wolf PA, Abbott RD, Kannel WB. Atrial fibrillation as an independent risk factor for stroke: The Framingham Study. Stroke. 1991;**22**:983-988. DOI: 10.1161/01.STR.22.8.983

[35] Tanne D, Haim M, Goldbourt U, Boyko V, Doolman R, Adler Y, Brunner D, Behar S, Sela BA. Prospective study of serum homocysteine and risk of ischemic stroke among patients with preexisting coronary heart disease. Stroke. 2003;**34**:632-636. DOI: 10.1161/01.STR.0000060203.58958.35

[36] Ansari R, Mahta A, Mallack E, Luo JJ. Hyperhomocysteinemia and neurologic disorders: A review. Journal of Clinical Neurology. 2014;**10**:281-288. DOI: 10.3988/jcn.2014.10.4.281

[37] Bazzano LA. Folic acid supplementation and cardiovascular disease: The state of the art. American Journal of the Medical Sciences. 2009;**338**:48-49. DOI: 10.1097/MAJ.0b013e3181aaefd6

[38] Kannel WB, McGee DL. Diabetes and cardiovascular disease: The Framingham Study. Journal of the American Medical Association. 1979;**241**:2035-2038. DOI: 10.1001/jama.1979.03290450033020

[39] Gaede P, Vedel P, Larsen N, Jensen GV, Parving HH, Pedersen O. Multifactorial intervention and cardiovascular disease in patients with type 2 diabetes. New England Journal of Medicine. 2003;**348**:383-393. DOI: 10.1056/NEJMoa021778

[40] Curb JD, Pressel SL, Cutler JA, Savage PJ, Applegate WB, Black H, Camel G, Davis BR, Frost PH, Gonzalez N, Guthrie G, Oberman A, Rutan GH, Stamler J. Effect of diuretic-based antihypertensive treatment on cardiovascular disease risk in older diabetic patients with isolated systolic hypertension. Systolic Hypertension in the Elderly Program Cooperative Research Group. Journal of the American Medical Association. 1996;**276**:1886-1892. Erratum in Journal of the American Medical Association. 1997, **277**:1356. DOI: 10.1001/jama.1996.03540230036032

[41] Iso H, Jacobs DR Jr, Wentworth D, Neaton JD, Cohen JD. Serum cholesterol levels and six-year mortality from stroke in 350,977 men screened for the multiple risk factor intervention trial. New England Journal of Medicine. 1989;**320**:904-910. DOI: 10.1056/NEJM198904063201405

[42] Kagan A, Popper JS, Rhoads GG. Factors related to stroke incidence in Hawaii Japanese men. The Honolulu Heart Study. Stroke. 1980;**11**:14-21. DOI: 10.1161/01.STR.11.1.14

[43] Leppala JM, Virtamo J, Fogelholm R, Albanes D, Heinoren OP. Different risk factors for different stroke subtypes: Association of blood pressure, cholesterol, and antioxidants. Stroke. 1999;**30**:2535-2540. DOI: 10.1161/01.STR.30.12.2535

[44] Gordon T, Kannel WB, Castelli WP, Dawber TR. Lipoproteins, cardiovascular disease, and death. The Framingham Study. Archives of Internal Medicine. 1981;**141**:1128-1131. DOI: 10.1001/archinte.1981.00340090024008

[45] Lindenstrom E, Boysen G, Nyboe J. Influence of total cholesterol, high density lipoprotein cholesterol, and triglycerides on risk of cerebrovascular disease: The Copenhagen City Heart Study. British Medical Journal. 1994;**309**:11-15. Erratum in British Medical Journal. 1994, **309**:1619

[46] Wannamethee SG, Shaper AG, Ebrahim S. HDL-cholesterol, total cholesterol, and the risk of stroke in middle-aged British men. Stroke. 2000;**31**:1882-1888. DOI: 10.1161/01.STR.31.8.1882

[47] Soyama Y, Miura K, Morikawa Y, Nishijo M, Nakanishi Y, Naruse Y, Kagamimori S, Nakagawa H. Oyabe Study. High-density lipoprotein cholesterol and risk of stroke in Japanese men and women: The Oyabe Study. Stroke. 2003;**34**:863-868. DOI: 10.1161/01.STR.0000060869.34009.38

[48] Collins R, Armitage J, Parish S, Sleight P, Peto R. Heart Protection Study Collaborative Group. Effects of cholesterol-lowering with simvastatin on stroke and other major vascular events in 20536 people with cerebrovascular disease or other high-risk conditions. Lancet. 2004;**363**:757-767. DOI: 10.1016/S0140-6736(04)15690-0

[49] Isozumi K. Obesity as a risk factor for cerebrovascular disease. Keio Journal of Medicine. 2004;**53**:7-11. DOI: 10.2302/kjm.53.7

[50] Boehme AK, Esenwa C, Elkind MS. Stroke Risk Factors, Genetics, and Prevention. Circulation Research. 2017;**120**:472-495. DOI: 10.1161/CIRCRESAHA.116.308398.

[51] Traylor M, Malik R, Nalls MA, Cotlarciuc I, Radmanesh F, Thorleifsson G, Hanscombe KB, Langefeld C, Saleheen D, Rost N, Yet I, Spector TD, Bell JT, Hannon E, Mill J, Chauhan G, Debette S, Bis JC, Longstreth WT Jr, Ikram MA, Launer LJ, Seshadri S. METASTROKE, UK Young Lacunar DNA Study, NINDS Stroke Genetics Network, Neurology Working Group of the CHARGE Consortium, Hamilton-Bruce MA, Jimenez-Conde J, Cole JW, Schmidt R, Słowik A, Lemmens R, Lindgren A, Melander O, Grewal RP, Sacco RL, Rundek T, Rexrode K, Arnett DK, Johnson JA, Benavente OR, Wasssertheil-Smoller S, Lee JM, Pulit SL, Wong Q, Rich SS, de Bakker PI, McArdle PF, Woo D, Anderson CD, Xu H, Heitsch L, Fornage M, Jern C, Stefansson K, Thorsteinsdottir U, Gretarsdottir S, Lewis CM, Sharma P, Sudlow CL, Rothwell PM, Boncoraglio GB, Thijs V, Levi C, Meschia JF, Rosand J, Kittner SJ, Mitchell BD, Dichgans M, Worrall BB, Markus HS. International Stroke Genetics Consortium. Genetic variation at 16q24.2 is associated with small vessel stroke. Annals of Neurology. 2017;**81**:383-394. DOI: 10.1002/ana.24840

[52] Kotlęga D, Peda B, Zembroń-Łacny A, Gołąb-Janowska M, Nowacki P. The role of brain-derived neurotrophic factor and its single nucleotide polymorphisms in stroke patients. Neurologia i Neurochirurgia Polska. 2017;**S0028-S3843**(16):30237-7. DOI: 10.1016/j.pjnns.2017.02.008. [Epub ahead of print]

[53] Hauser WA, Annegers JF, Kurland LT. Incidence of epilepsy and unprovoked seizures in Rochester, Minnesota: 1935-1984. Epilepsia. 1993;**34**:453-468

[54] Olafsson E, Ludvigsson P, Gudmundsson G, Hesdorffer D, Kjartansson O, Hauser WA. Incidence of unprovoked seizures and epilepsy in Iceland and assessment of the epilepsy syndrome classification: A prospective study. Lancet Neurology. 2005;**4**:627-634. DOI: 10.1016/S1474-4422(05)70172-1

[55] Jędrzejczak J. Epilepsy. The hardest are the answers to simple questions. Termedia, Poznań; 2008; 6-11. Book In Polish

[56] Fernandez-Torre JL, Rebollo M. Typical absence status epilepticus as late presentation of idiopathic generalised epilepsy in an elderly patient. Seizure. 2009;**18**:82-83. DOI: 10.1016/j.seizure.2008.08.005

[57] Ramsay RE, Rowan AJ, Pryor FM. Special considerations in treating the elderly patient with epilepsy. Neurology. 2004;**62**:24-29

[58] Pugh MJ, Knoefel JE, Mortensen EM, Amuan ME, Berlowitz DR, Van Cott AC. New-onset epilepsy risk factors in older veterans. Journal of the American Geriatrics Society. 2009;**57**:237-242. DOI: 10.1111/j.1532-5415.2008.02124.x

[59] Stephen LJ, Brodie MJ. Epilepsy in elderly people. Lancet. 2000;**355**:1441-1446. DOI: 10.1016/S0140-6736(00)02149-8

[60] Tanaka A, Akamatsu N, Shouzaki T, Toyota T, Yamano M, Nakagawa M, Tsuji S. Clinical characteristics and treatment responses in new-onset epilepsy in the elderly. Seizure. 2013;**22**:772-775. DOI: 10.1016/j.seizure.2013.06.005

[61] Assis TM, Bacellar A, Costa G, Nascimento OJ. Mortality predictors of epilepsy and epileptic seizures among hospitalized elderly. Arquivos de Neuro-psiquiatria. 2015;**73**:510-515. DOI: 10.1590/0004-282X20150043

[62] Alberti A, Paciaroni M, Caso V, Venti M, Palmerini F, Agnelli G. Early seizures in patients with acute stroke: Frequency, predictive factors, and effect on clinical outcome. Vascular Health Risk Management. 2008;**4**:715-720

[63] Renu A, Amaro S, Laredo C, Román LS, Llull L, Lopez A, Urra X, Blasco J, Oleaga L, Chamorro Á. Relevance of blood-brain barrier disruption after endovascular treatment of ischemic stroke: Dual-energy computed tomographic study. Stroke. 2015;**46**:673-679. DOI: 10.1161/STROKEAHA.114.008147

[64] Yang H, Song Z, Yang GP, Zhang BK, Chen M, Wu T, Guo R. The ALDH2 rs671 polymorphism affects poststroke epilepsy susceptibility and plasma 4-HNE levels. PLoS One. 2014;**10**:e109634. DOI: 10.1371/journal.pone.0109634

[65] Zhang B, Chen M, Yang H, Wu T, Song C, Guo R. Evidence for involvement of the CD40/CD40L system in poststroke epilepsy. Neuroscience Letters. 2014;**567**:6-10. DOI: 10.1016/j.neulet.2014.03.003

[66] Pitkänen A, Roivainen R, Lukasiuk K. Development of epilepsy after ischaemic stroke. Lancet Neurology. 2006;**15**:185-197. DOI: 10.1016/S1474-4422(15)00248-3

[67] Annegers JF, Hauser WA, Coan SP, Rocca WA. A population-based study of seizures after traumatic brain injuries. New England Journal of Medicine. 1998;**338**:20-24. DOI: 10.1056/NEJM199801013380104

[68] Diaz-Arrastia R, Gong Y, Fair S, Scott KD, Garcia MC, Carlile MC, Agostini MA, Van Ness PC. Increased risk of late posttraumatic seizures associated with inheritance of APOE epsilon4 allele. Archives of Neurology. 2003;**60**:818-822. DOI: 10.1001/archneur.60.6.818

[69] Assis TR, Bacellar A, Costa G, Nascimento OJ. Etiological prevalence of epilepsy and epileptic seizures in hospitalized elderly in a Brazilian tertiary center-Salvador—Brazil. Arquivos de Neuro-psiquiatria. 2015;**73**:83-89. DOI: 10.1590/0004-282X20140217

[70] Maschio M. Brain tumor-related epilepsy. Current Neuropharmacology. 2012;**10**:124-133. DOI: 10.2174/157015912800604470

[71] Petras M, Tatarkova Z, Kovalska M, Mokra D, Dobrota D, Lehotsky J, Drgova A. Hyperhomocysteinemia as a risk factor for the neuronal system disorders. Journal of Physiology and Pharmacology: An official Journal of the Polish Physiological Society. 2014;**65**:15-23

[72] Marszałł ML, Makarowski R, Hinc S, Kłos M, Czarnowski W. Hyperhomocysteinemia in active and passive smokers and the levels of folate and vitamin B6 in plasma. Przegląd Lekarski. 2008;**65**:486-490. In Polish

[73] Cravo ML, Camilo ME. Hyperhomocysteinemia in chronic alcoholism: relations to folic acid and vitamins B(6) and B(12) status. Nutrition. 2000;**16**:296-302

[74] Tomaszewski J, Pieprzowska-Białek A, Skorupski P, Rechberger T. Elevated serum homocysteine concentration in women taking oral hormone replacement therapy. Przegląd Menopauzalny. 2003;**5**:31-34. In Polish

[75] Dorszewska J, Winczewska-Wiktor A, Sniezawska A, Kaczmarek I, Steinborn B. Homocysteine and asymmetric dimethylarginine (ADMA) in epilepsy. Przegląd Lekarski. 2009, **8**:448-452. In Polish

[76] Schwaninger M, Ringleb P, Winter R, Kohl B, Fiehn W, Rieser PA, Walter-Sack I. Elevated plasma concentrations of homocysteine in antiepileptic drug treatment. Epilepsia. 1999, **40**:345-350

[77] Ghosh S, Jehi LE. New-onset epilepsy in the elderly: Challenges for the internist. Cleveland Clinic Journal of Medicine. 2014;**81**:490-498. DOI: 10.3949/ccjm.81a.13148

[78] Krämer G. Epilepsy in the Elderly: Some clinical and pharmacotherapeutic aspects. Epilepsia. 2001;**42**:55-59

[79] N'Gouemo P. Altered voltage-gated calcium channels in rat inferior colliculus neurons contribute to alcohol withdrawal seizures. European Neuropsychopharmacology. 2015;**25**:1342-1352. DOI: 10.1016/j.euroneuro.2015.04.008

[80] Imfeld P, Bodmer M, Schuerch M, Jick SS, Meier CR. Seizures in patients with Alzheimer's disease or vascular dementia: A population-based nested case-control analysis. Epilepsia. 2013;**54**:700-707. DOI: 10.1111/epi.12045

[81] Amatniek JC, Hauser WA, DelCastillo-Castaneda C, Jacobs DM, Marder K, Bell K, Albert M, Brandt J, Stern Y. Incidence and predictors of seizures in patients with Alzheimer's disease. Epilepsia. 2006;**47**:867-872

[82] Bernardi S, Scaldaferri N, Vanacore N, Trebbastoni A, Francia A, D'Amico A, Prencipe M. Seizures in Alzheimer's disease: A retrospective study of a cohort of outpatients. Epileptic Disorders. 2010;**12**:16-21. DOI: 10.1684/epd.2010.0290

[83] Rao SC, Dove G, Cascino GD, Petersen RC. Recurrent seizures in patients with dementia: Frequency, seizure types, and treatment outcome. Epilepsy & Behavior. 2009;**14**:118-120. DOI: 10.1016/j.yebeh.2008.08.012

[84] Irizarry MC, Jin S, He F, Emond JA, Raman R, Thomas RG, Sano M, Quinn JF, Tariot PN, Galasko DR, Ishihara LS, Weil JG, Aisen PS. Incidence of new-onset seizures in mild to moderate Alzheimer disease. Archives of Neurology. 2012;**69**:368-372. DOI: 10.1001/archneurol.2011.830

[85] Roberson ED, Hope OA, Martin RC, Schmidt D. Geriatric epilepsy: Research and clinical directions for the future. Epilepsy & Behavior. 2011;**22**:103-111. DOI: 10.1016/j.yebeh.2011.04.005

[86] Etemadifar M, Abtahi SH, Minagar A, Akbari M, Masaeli A, Tabrizi N. Late-onset multiple sclerosis in Isfahan, Iran. Archives of Iran Medicine. 2012;**15**:596-598. DOI: 0121510/AIM.004

[87] Sponsler JL, Kendrick-Adey AC. Seizures as a manifestation of multiple sclerosis. Epileptic Disorders. 2011;**13**:401-410. DOI: 10.1684/epd.2011.0468

[88] Allen AN, Seminog OO, Goldacre MJ. Association between multiple sclerosis and epilepsy: Large population-based record-linkage studies. BMC Neurology. 2013;**13**:189. DOI: 10.1186/1471-2377-13-189

[89] Viveiros CD, Alvarenga RM. Prevalence of epilepsy in a case series of multiple sclerosis patients. Arquivos de Neuro-Psiquiatria. 2010;**68**:731-736

[90] Dorszewska J, Prendecki M, Oczkowska A, Dezor M, Kozubski W. Molecular basis of familial and sporadic Alzheimer's disease. Current Alzheimer Research. 2016;**13**:952-963. DOI: 10.2174/1567205013666160314150501

[91] Hachinski VC, Lassen NA, Marshall J. Multi-infarct dementia. A cause of mental deterioration in the elderly. Lancet. 1974;**2**:207-210

[92] Hachinski VC, Bowler JV. Vascular dementia. Neurology. 1993;**43**:2159-2160

[93] O'Brien JT, Erkinjuntti T, Reisberg B, Roman G, Sawada T, Pantoni L, Bowler JV, Ballard C, DeCarli C, Gorelick PB, Rockwood K, Burns A, Gauthier S, DeKosky ST. Vascular cognitive impairment. Lancet Neurology. 2003;**2**:89-98. DOI: 10.1016/S1474-4422(03)00305-3

[94] Lobo A, Launer LJ, Fratiglioni L, Andersen K, Di Carlo A, Breteler MM, Copeland JR, Dartigues JF, Jagger C, Martinez-Lage J, Soininen H, Hofman A. Prevalence of dementia and major subtypes in Europe: A collaborative study of population-based cohorts. Neurologic Diseases in the Elderly Research Group. Neurology. 2000;**54**:S4-S9

[95] Fratiglioni L, Launer LJ, Andersen K, Breteler MM, Copeland JR, Dartigues JF, Lobo A, Martinez-Lage J, Soininen H, Hofman A. Incidence of dementia and major subtypes in Europe: A collaborative study of population-based cohorts. Neurologic Diseases in the Elderly Research Group. Neurology. 2000;**54**:S10-S15

[96] Hébert R, Brayne C. Epidemiology of vascular dementia. Neuroepidemiology. 1995; **14**:240-257

[97] Rockwood K, Wentzel C, Hachinski V, Hogan DB, MacKnight C, McDowell I. Prevalence and outcomes of vascular cognitive impairment. Vascular Cognitive Impairment Investigators of the Canadian Study of Health and Aging. Neurology. 2000;**54**:447-451

[98] Jorm AF, Jolley D. The incidence of dementia: A meta-analysis. Neurology. 1998;**51**:728-733

[99] Ukraintseva S, Sloan F, Arbeev K, Yashin A. Increasing rates of dementia at time of declining mortality from stroke. Stroke. 2006;**37**:1155-115915. DOI: 10.1161/01.STR.0000217971.88034.e9

[100] Hébert R, Lindsay J, Verreault R, Rockwood K, Hill G, Dubois MF. Vascular dementia: Incidence and risk factors in the Canadian study of health and aging. Stroke. 2000;**31**:1487-1493. DOI: 10.1161/01.STR.31.7.1487

[101] Kuller LH, Lopez OL, Jagust WJ, Becker JT, DeKosky ST, Lyketsos C, Kawas C, Breitner JC, Fitzpatrick A, Dulberg C. Determinants of vascular dementia in the Cardiovascular Health Cognition Study. Neurology. 2005;**64**:1548-1582

[102] Suryadevara V, Storey SG, Aronow WS, Ahn C. Association of abnormal serum lipids in elderly persons with atherosclerotic vascular disease and dementia, atherosclerotic vascular disease without dementia, dementia without atherosclerotic vascular disease, and no dementia or atherosclerotic vascular disease. The Journals of Gerontology. Series A, Biological Sciences and Medical Sciences. 2003;**58**:M859-M861

[103] Reitz C, Tang MX, Luchsinger J, Mayeux R. Relation of plasma lipids to Alzheimer disease and vascular dementia. Archives of Neurology. 2004;**61**:705-714. DOI: 10.1001/archneur.61.5.705

[104] Posner HB, Tang MX, Luchsinger J, Antigua R, Stern Y, Mayeux R. The relationship of hypertension in the elderly to AD, vascular dementia, and cognitive function. Neurology. 2002;**58**:1175-1181

[105] Ross GW, Petrovitch H, White LR, Masaki KH, Li CY, Curb JD, Yano K, Rodriguez BL, Foley DJ, Blanchette PL, Havlik R. Characterization of risk factors for vascular dementia: The Honolulu-Asia Aging Study. Neurology. 1999;**53**:337-343

[106] Ott A, Stolk RP, Hofman A, van Harskamp F, Grobbee DE, Breteler MM. Association of diabetes mellitus and dementia: the Rotterdam Study. Diabetologia. 1996;**39**:1392-1397

[107] Geroldi C, Frisoni GB, Paolisso G, Bandinelli S, Lamponi M, Abbatecola AM, Zanetti O, Guralnik JM, Ferrucci L. Insulin resistance in cognitive impairment: the InCHIANTI study. Archives of Neurology. 2005;**62**:1067-1072. DOI: 10.1001/archneur.62.7.1067

[108] Ahtiluoto S, Polvikoski T, Peltonen M, Solomon A, Tuomilehto J, Winblad B, Sulkava R, Kivipelto M. Diabetes, Alzheimer disease, and vascular dementia: A population-based neuropathologic study. Neurology. 2010'**75**:1195-1202. DOI: 10.1212/WNL.0b013e3181f4d7f8

[109] Dichgans M, Zietemann V. Prevention of vascular cognitive impairment. Stroke. 2012;**43**:3137-3146. DOI: 10.1161/STROKEAHA.112.651778

[110] Kalmijn S, Foley D, White L, Burchfiel CM, Curb JD, Petrovitch H, Ross GW, Havlik RJ, Launer LJ. Metabolic cardiovascular syndrome and risk of dementia in Japanese-American elderly men. The Honolulu-Asia aging study. Arteriosclerosis, Thrombosis, and Vascular Biology. 2000;**20**:2255-2260. DOI: 10.1161/01.ATV.20.10.2255

[111] Solfrizzi V, Scafato E, Capurso C, D'Introno A, Colacicco AM, Frisardi V, Vendemiale G, Baldereschi M, Crepaldi G, Di Carlo A, Galluzzo L, Gandin C, Inzitari D, Maggi S, Capurso A, Panza F. Italian Longitudinal Study on Ageing Working Group. Metabolic syndrome and the risk of vascular dementia: The Italian Longitudinal Study on Ageing. Journal of Neurology, Neurosurgery and Psychiatry. 2010;**81**:433-440. DOI: 10.1136/jnnp.2009.181743

[112] Segura B, Jurado MA, Freixenet N, Albuin C, Muniesa J, Junqué C. Mental slowness and executive dysfunctions in patients with metabolic syndrome. Neuroscience Letters. 2009;**462**:49-53. DOI: 10.1016/j.neulet.2009.06.071

[113] Newman GC, Bang H, Hussain SI, Toole JF. Association of diabetes, homocysteine, and HDL with cognition and disability after stroke. Neurology. 2007;**69**:2054-2062

[114] Ivan CS, Seshadri S, Beiser A, Au R, Kase CS, Kelly-Hayes M, Wolf PA. Dementia after stroke: The Framingham Study. Stroke. 2004;**35**:1264-1268. DOI: 10.1161/01.STR.0000127810.92616.78

[115] Desmond DW, Moroney JT, Sano M, Stern Y. Incidence of dementia after ischemic stroke: Results of a longitudinal study. Stroke. 2002;**33**:2254-2260. DOI: 10.1161/01.STR.0000028235.91778.95

[116] Altieri M, Di Piero V, Pasquini M, Gasparini M, Vanacore N, Vicenzini E, Lenzi GL. Delayed poststroke dementia: a 4-year follow-up study. Neurology. 2004;**62**:2193-2197

[117] Lin JH, Lin RT, Tai CT, Hsieh CL, Hsiao SF, Liu CK. Prediction of poststroke dementia. Neurology. 2003;**61**:343-348

[118] Censori B, Manara O, Agostinis C, Camerlingo M, Casto L, Galavotti B, Partziguian T, Servalli MC, Cesana B, Belloni G, Mamoli A. Dementia after first stroke. Stroke. 1996;**27**:1205-1210. DOI: 10.1161/01.STR.27.7.1205

[119] Inzitari D, Di Carlo A, Pracucci G, Lamassa M, Vanni P, Romanelli M, Spolveri S, Adriani P, Meucci I, Landini G, Ghetti A. Incidence and determinants of poststroke dementia as defined by an informant interview method in a hospital-based stroke registry. Stroke. 1998;**29**:2087-2093. DOI: 10.1161/01.STR.29.10.2087

[120] Pohjasvaara T, Erkinjuntti T, Ylikoski R, Hietanen M, Vataja R, Kaste M. Clinical determinants of poststroke dementia. Stroke. 1998;**29**:75-81. DOI: 10.1161/01.STR.29.1.75

[121] Kokmen E, Whisnant JP, O'Fallon WM, Chu CP, Beard CM. Dementia after ischemic stroke: A population-based study in Rochester, Minnesota (1960-1984). Neurology. 1996;**46**:154-159

[122] Srikanth VK, Quinn SJ, Donnan GA, Saling MM, Thrift AG. Long-term cognitive transitions, rates of cognitive change, and predictors of incident dementia in a population-based first-ever stroke cohort. Stroke. 2006;**37**:2479-2483. DOI: 10.1161/01.STR.0000239666.46828.d7

[123] Leys D, Hénon H, Mackowiak-Cordoliani MA, Pasquier F. Poststroke dementia. Lancet Neurology. 2005;**4**:752-759. DOI: 10.1016/S1474-4422(05)70221-0

[124] Melkas S, Oksala NK, Jokinen H, Pohjasvaara T, Vataja R, Oksala A, Kaste M, Karhunen PJ, Erkinjuntti T. Poststroke dementia predicts poor survival in long-term follow-up: Influence of prestroke cognitive decline and previous stroke. Journal of Neurology, Neurosurgery, and Psychiatry. 2009;**80**:865-870. DOI: 10.1136/jnnp.2008.166603

[125] Gottesman RF, Hillis AE. Predictors and assessment of cognitive dysfunction resulting from ischaemic stroke. Lancet Neurology. 2010;**9**:895-905. DOI: 10.1016/S1474-4422(10)70164-2

[126] Béjot Y, Aboa-Eboulé C, Durier J, Rouaud O, Jacquin A, Ponavoy E, Richard D, Moreau T, Giroud M. Prevalence of early dementia after first-ever stroke: A 24-year population-based study. Stroke. 2011;**42**:607-612. DOI: 10.1161/STROKEAHA.110.595553

[127] Dong Y, Venketasubramanian N, Chan BP, Sharma VK, Slavin MJ, Collinson SL, Sachdev P, Chan YH, Chen CL. Brief screening tests during acute admission in patients with mild stroke are predictive of vascular cognitive impairment 3-6 months after stroke. Journal of Neurology Neurosurgery, and Psychiatry. 2012;**83**:580-585. DOI: 10.1136/jnnp-2011-302070

[128] Rist PM, Chalmers J, Arima H, Sharma VK, Slavin MJ, Collinson SL, Sachdev P, Chan YH, Chen CL. Baseline cognitive function, recurrent stroke, and risk of dementia in patients with stroke. Stroke. 2013;**44**:1790-1795. DOI: 10.1136/jnnp-2011-302070

[129] Gamaldo A, Moghekar A, Kilada S, Resnick SM, Zonderman AB, O'Brien R. Effect of a clinical stroke on the risk of dementia in a prospective cohort. Neurology. 2006;**67**:1363-1369. DOI: 10.1212/01.wnl.0000240285.89067.3f

[130] Narasimhalu K, Ang S, De Silva DA, Wong MC, Chang HM, Chia KS, Auchus AP, Chen C. Severity of CIND and MCI predict incidence of dementia in an ischemic stroke cohort. Neurology. 2009;**73**:1866-1872. DOI: 10.1212/WNL.0b013e3181c3fcb7

[131] Wang Q, Capistrant BD, Ehntholt A, Glymour MM. Long-term rate of change in memory functioning before and after stroke onset. Stroke. 2012;**43**:2561-2566. DOI: 10.1161/STROKEAHA.112.661587

[132] Prendecki M, Florczak-Wyspianska J, Kowalska M, Lianeri M, Kozubski W, Dorszewska J. Normal aging and dementia. Davide M, editor. In: Update on Dementia. InTech, Rijeka; 2016; 251-272. DOI: 10.5772/64203

[133] Selkoe DJ. Alzheimer's disease: Genes, proteins, and therapy. Physiological Reviews. 2001;**81**:741-766

[134] Alonso Vilatela ME, López-López M, Yescas-Gómez P. Genetics of Alzheimer's disease. Archives of Medical Research. 2012;**43**:622-631. DOI: 10.1016/j.arcmed.2012.10.017

[135] Lambert JC, Ibrahim-Verbaas CA, Harold D, Naj AC, Sims R, Bellenguez C, et al. Meta-analysis of 74,046 individuals identifies 11 new susceptibility loci for Alzheimer's disease. Nature Genetics. 2013. **45**:1452-1458. DOI: 10.1038/ng.2802

[136] http://www.alzgene.org/- date of access 02.03.2017

[137] McKhann GM, Knopman DS, Chertkow H, Hyman BT, Jack CR Jr, Kawas CH, Klunk WE, Koroshetz WJ, Manly JJ, Mayeux R, Mohs RC, Morris JC, Rossor MN, Scheltens P, Carrillo MC, Thies B, Weintraub S, Phelps CH. The diagnosis of dementia due to Alzheimer's disease: Recommendations from the National Institute on Aging-Alzheimer's Association workgroups on diagnostic guidelines for Alzheimer's disease. Alzheimers and Dementia. 2011;**7**:263-269. DOI: 10.1016/j.jalz.2011.03.005

[138] Martin E, Boucher C, Fontaine B, Delarasse C. Distinct inflammatory phenotypes of microglia and monocyte-derived macrophages in Alzheimer's disease models: Effects of aging and amyloid pathology. Aging Cell. 2017;**16**:27-38. DOI: 10.1111/acel.12522

[139] Zhang ZG, Li Y, Ng CT, Song YQ. Inflammation in Alzheimer's disease and molecular genetics: Recent update. Archivum Immunologiae et Therapiae Experimentalis. 2015;**63**:333-344. DOI: 10.1007/s00005-015-0351-0

[140] Parsons CG, Danysz W, Dekundy A, Pulte I. Memantine and cholinesterase inhibitors: Complementary mechanisms in the treatment of Alzheimer's disease. Neurotoxicity Research. 2013;**24**:358-369. DOI: 10.1007/s12640-013-9398-z

[141] Mendiola-Precoma J, Berumen LC, Padilla K, Garcia-Alcocer G. Therapies for prevention and treatment of Alzheimer's disease. Biomed Research International. 2016;**2016**:2589276. DOI: 10.1155/2016/2589276

[142] Dolejší E, Liraz O, Rudajev V, Zimčík P, Doležal V, Michaelson DM. Apolipoprotein E4 reduces evoked hippocampal acetylcholine release in adult mice. Journal of Neurochemistry. 2016;**136**:503-509. DOI: 10.1111/jnc.13417

[143] Reeve A, Simcox E, Turnbull D. Ageing and Parkinson's disease: Why is advancing age the biggest risk factor? Ageing Research Reviews. 2014;**14**:19-30. DOI: 10.1016/j.arr.2014.01.004

[144] Tata A, Velluto L, D'Angelo C, Reale M. Cholinergic system dysfunction and neurodegenerative diseases: Cause or effect? CNS and Neurological Disorders Drug Targets. 2014;**13**:1294-1303. DOI: 10.2174/1871527313666140917121132

[145] Troesch B, Weber P, Mohajeri MH. Potential links between impaired one-carbon metabolism due to polymorphisms, inadequate B-vitamin status, and the development of Alzheimer's disease. Nutrients. 2016;**8**:E803. DOI: 10.3390/nu8120803

[146] Hughes AJ, Daniel SE, Kilford L, Lees AJ. Accuracy of clinical diagnosis of idiopathic Parkinson's disease: A clinico-pathological study of 100 cases. Journal of Neurology, Neurosurgery and Psychiatry. 1992;**55**:181-184. DOI: 10.1136/jnnp.55.3.181

[147] Dorszewska J, Kozubski W. Introductory chapter—genetic and biochemical factors in Parkinson's disease. Dorszewska J, Kozubski W, editors. In: Challenges in Parkinson's disease. InTech, Rijeka; 2016; 1-6. DOI: 10.5772/61880

[148] Przedborski S, Jackson-Lewis V. Mechanisms of MPTP toxicity. Movement Disorders. 1998;**13**:35-38

[149] Nagatsu T, Mogi M, Ichinose H, Togari A. Changes in cytokines and neurotrophins in Parkinson's disease. Journal of Neural Transmission. 2000;**60**(Supplementum): 277-290

[150] Bartels AL, Leenders KL. Cyclooxygenase and neuroinflammation in Parkinson's disease neurodegeneration. Current Neuropharmacology. 2010;**8**:62-68. DOI: 10.2174/157015 910790909485

[151] Litteljohn D, Mangano E, Clarke M, Bobyn J, Moloney K, Hayley S. Inflammatory mechanisms of neurodegeneration in toxin-based models of Parkinson's disease. Parkinson's Disease. 2011;**2010**:713517. DOI:10.4061/2011/713517

[152] Goldman SM. Environmental toxins and Parkinson's disease. Annual Review of Pharmacology and Toxicology. 2014;**54**:141-164. DOI: 10.1146/annurev-pharmtox-011613-135937

[153] Golts N, Snyder H, Frasier M, Theisler C, Choi P, Wolozin B. Magnesium inhibits spontaneous and iron-induced aggregation of alpha-synuclein. Journal of Biological Chemistry. 2002;**277**:16116-16123. DOI: 10.1074/jbc.M107866200

[154] Bartzokis G, Tishler TA, Shin IS, Lu PH, Cummings JL. Brain ferritin iron as a risk factor for age at onset in neurodegenerative diseases. Annals of the New York Academy of Sciences. 2004;**1012**:224-236. DOI: 10.1196/annals.1306.019

[155] Oczkowska A, Kozubski W, Lianeri M, Dorszewska J. Genetic variants in diseases of the extrapyramidal system. Current Genomics. 2014;**15**:18-27. DOI: 10.2174/138920291 4666131210213327

[156] Dorszewska J, Kowalska M, Blaszczak W, Kozubski W. Molecular basis of neurodegeneration in Parkinson's disease. In: Neurodegenerative Diseases: Overview, Perspectives and Emerging Treatment. NY, USA: NOVA Sciences Publishers, Inc; 2017. [in press].

[157] Raver SM, & Lin S-C. Basal forebrain motivational salience signal enhances cortical processing and decision speed. Frontiers of Behavioral Neuroscience. 2015;**9**:eCollection 2015. DOI: 10.3389/fnbeh.2015.00277

[158] Hirsch EC, Graybiel AM, Duyckaerts C, Javoy-Agid F. Neuronal loss in the pedunculopontine tegmental nucleus in Parkinson disease and in progressive supranuclear palsy. Proceedings of the National Academy of Sciences. 1987;**84**:5976-5980

[159] Buchman AS, Shulman JM, Nag S, Leurgans SE, Arnold SE, Morris MC, Schneider JA, Bennett DA. Nigral pathology and parkinsonian signs in elders without Parkinson disease. Annals of Neurology. 2012;**71**:258-266. DOI: 10.1002/ana.22588

[160] Horvath S, Ritz BR. Increased epigenetic age and granulocyte counts in the blood of Parkinson's disease patients. Aging (Albany NY). 2015;**7**:1130-1142. DOI: 10.18632/aging.100859

[161] Matsumoto L, Takuma H, Tamaoka A, Kurisaki H, Date H, Tsuji S, Iwata A. CpG demethylation enhances alpha-synuclein expression and affects the pathogenesis of Parkinson's disease. PLoS One. 2010;**5**:e15522. DOI: 10.1371/journal.pone.0015522

[162] Goers J, Manning-Bog AB, McCormack AL, Millett IS, Doniach S, Di Monte DA, Uversky VN, Fink AL. Nuclear localization of alpha-synuclein and its interaction with histones. Biochemistry. 2003;**42**:8465-8471. DOI: 10.1021/bi0341152

[163] Elahy M, Jackaman C, Mamo JC, Lam V, Dhaliwal SS, Giles C, Nelson D, Takechi R. Blood–brain barrier dysfunction developed during normal aging is associated with inflammation and loss of tight junctions but not with leukocyte recruitment. Immunity and Ageing. 2015;**12**:2. DOI: 10.1186/s12979-015-0029-9

[164] Cabezas R, Avila M, Gonzalez J, El-Bachá RS, Báez E, García-Segura LM, Jurado Coronel JC, Capani F, Cardona-Gomez GP, Barreto GE. Astrocytic modulation of blood brain barrier: Perspectives on Parkinson's disease. Frontiers in Cellular Neuroscience. 2014;**8**:211. DOI: 10.3389/fncel.2014.00211

[165] Białecka M, Kurzawski M, Roszmann A, Robowski P, Sitek EJ, Honczarenko K, Gorzkowska A, Budrewicz S, Mak M, Jarosz M, Gołąb-Janowska M, Koziorowska-Gawron E, Droździk M, Sławek J. Association of COMT, MTHFR, and SLC19A1(RFC-1) polymorphisms with homocysteine blood levels and cognitive impairment in Parkinson's disease. Pharmacogenetics Genomics. 2012;**22**:716-724. DOI: 10.1097/FPC.0b013e32835693f7

[166] Białecka M, Robowski P, Honczarenko K, Roszmann A, Sławek J. Genetic and environmental factors for hyperhomocysteinaemia and its clinical implications in Parkinson's disease. Polish Neurology and Neurosurgery. 2009;**43**:272-285. In Polish

[167] Zoccolella S, Lamberti P, Armenise E, de Mari M, Lamberti SV, Mastronardi R, Fraddosio A, Iliceto G, Livrea P. Plasma homocysteine levels in Parkinson's disease: Role of antiparkinsonian medications. Parkinsonism and Related Disorders. 2005;**11**:131-133. DOI: 10.1016/j.parkreldis.2004.07.008

[168] Mattson MP, Shea TB. Folate and homocysteine metabolism in neural plasticity and neurodegenerative disorders. Trends in Neurosciences. 2003;**26**:137-146. DOI: 10.1016/S0166-2236(03)00032-8

[169] Louis DN, Perry A, Reifenberger G, von Deimling A, Figarella-Branger D, Cavenee WK, Ohgaki H, Wiestler OD, Kleihues P, Ellison DW. The 2016 World Health Organization Classification of tumors of the central nervous system: A summary. Acta Neuropathologica. 2016;**131**:803-820. DOI: 10.1007/s00401-016-1545-1

[170] Lorimer CF, Saran F, Chalmers AJ, Brock J. Glioblastoma in the elderly — How do we choose who to treat?. Journal of Geriatric Oncology. 2016;**7**:453-456. DOI: 10.1016/j.jgo.2016.07.005

[171] Mohile NA. How I treat glioblastoma in older patients. Journal of Geriatric Oncology. 2016;**7**:1-6. DOI: 10.1016/j.jgo.2015.12.001

[172] Schneider T, Mawrin C, Scherlach C, Skalej M, Firsching R. Gliomas in adults. Deutsches Arzteblat International. 2010;**107**:799-807. quiz 808. DOI: 10.3238/arztebl.2010.0799

[173] Scott JG, Bauchet L, Fraum TJ, Nayak L, Cooper AR, Chao ST, Suh JH, Vogelbaum MA, Peereboom DM, Zouaoui S, Mathieu-Daude H, Fabbro-Peray P, Rigau V, Tailandier L, Abrey LE, DeAngelis LM, Shih JH, Iwamoto FM. Recursive partitioning analysis of prognostic factors for glioblastoma patients aged 70 years or older. Cancer. 2012;**118**:5595-5600. DOI: 10.1002/cncr.27570

[174] Rampling R, Erridge S. Management of Central Nervous System Tumours in the elderly. Clinical Oncology (Royal College of Radiologists (Great Britain)). 2014;**26**:431-437. DOI: 10.1016/j.clon.2014.03.009

[175] Schittenhelm J, Skardelly M. Molecular advances In Glioblastoma Neuropathology. Agrawa A, editor. In: Neurooncology–Newer Developments. InTech, Rijeka; 2016; 3-26 DOI: 10.5772/62670

[176] Ahmed R, Oborski MJ, Hwang M, Lieberman FS, Mountz JM. Malignant gliomas: Current perspectives in diagnosis, treatment, and early response assessment using advanced quantitative imaging methods. Cancer Management and Research. 2014;**6**:149-170. DOI: 10.2147/CMAR.S54726

[177] Verhaak RGW, Hoadley KA, Purdom E, Wang V, Qi Y, Wilkerson MD, Miller CR, Ding L, Golub T, Mesirov JP, Alexe G, Lawrence M, O'Kelly M, Tamayo P, Weir BA, Gabriel S, Winckler W, Gupta S, Jakkula L, Feiler HS, Hodgson JG, James CD, Sarkaria JN, Brennan C, Kahn A, Spellman PT, Wilson RK, Speed TP, Gray JW, Meyerson M, Perou CM, Hayes DN, Cancer Genome Atlas Research Network, The Cancer Genome Atlas Research, Cancer Genome Atlas Research Network TCGAR. Integrated genomic analysis identifies clinically relevant subtypes of glioblastoma characterized by abnormalities in PDGFRA, IDH1, EGFR, and NF1. Cancer Cell. 2010, **17**:98-110. DOI: 10.1016/j.ccr.2009.12.020

[178] Flowers A. Brain tumors in the older person. Cancer Control: Journal of the Moffitt Cancer Center. 2000;**7**:523-538

[179] Jordan JT, Gerstner ER, Batchelor TT, Cahill DP, Plotkin SR. Glioblastoma care in the elderly. Cancer. 2016;**122**:189-197. DOI: 10.1002/cncr.29742

[180] Kita D, Ciernik IF, Vaccarella S, Franceschi S, Kleihues P, Lütolf UM, Ohgaki H. Age as a predictive factor in glioblastomas: Population-based study. Neuroepidemiology. 2009;**33**:17-22. DOI: 10.1159/000210017

[181] Narita Y. Bevacizumab for glioblastoma. Therapeutics and Clinical Risk Management. 2015;**11**:1759-1765. DOI: 10.2147/TCRM.S58289

[182] Cohen AL, Colman H. Glioma biology and molecular markers. Cancer Treatment and Research. 2015;**163**:15-30. DOI: 10.1007/978-3-319-12048-5_2

[183] Wirsching H-G, Galanis E, Weller M. Glioblastoma. Handbook of Clinical Neurology. 2016;**134**:381-397. DOI: 10.1016/B978-0-12-802997-8.00023-2

[184] Specenier P. Bevacizumab in glioblastoma multiforme. Expert Review on Anticancer Therapy. 2012;**12**:9-18. DOI: 10.1586/era.11.179

[185] Nghiemphu PL, Liu W, Lee Y, Than T, Graham C, Lai A, Green RM, Pope WB, Liau LM, Mischein PS, Nelson SF, Elashoff R, Cloughesy TF. Bevacizumab and chemotherapy for recurrent glioblastoma: A single-institution experience. Neurology. 2009;**72**:1217-1222. DOI: 10.1212/01.wnl.0000345668.03039.90

[186] Ohgaki H. Genetic pathways to glioblastomas. Neuropathology. 2005;**25**:1-7. DOI: 10.1111/j.1440-1789.2004.00600.x

Chapter 6

Presenilins Interactome in Alzheimer's Disease and Pathological Ageing

Michalina Maria Wężyk and Cezary Żekanowski

Additional information is available at the end of the chapter

http://dx.doi.org/10.5772/intechopen.68748

Abstract

Alzheimer's disease (AD) is the most common type of dementia characterized by massive neuronal loss. Pathological hallmarks of the disease are overproduction of β-amyloid (Aβ) and hyperphosphorylation of tau protein accumulated into senile plaques (SPs) and neurofibrillary tangles (NFTs), respectively. SPs with cortical tau pathology are also hallmark of pathological ageing (PA). Recently, an extensive overlap has been shown between Aβ levels and profiles in PA and AD brains, suggesting that PA could be a prodromal AD phase. Presenilins are major components of the γ-secretase complex involved in Aβ production. Furthermore, presenilins interact with players of numerous signalling pathways important in the PA and AD. Integration of various modern research approaches would reinforce the role of presenilins signalling network in brain pathology. These approaches include high-throughput (epi)genetic and transcriptomic analyses, large-scale microscopic imaging studies, immunoaffinity purification or mass spectrometry. Comprehensive integration of these methods is necessary to update the definition of the role of presenilins in AD and PA. Hereby, we summarize the available data on presenilins' functions and interactions. We believe that the systematization of the existing knowledge will stimulate further research and will help reveal the molecular nooks and crannies in Alzheimer's disease and in pathological ageing.

Keywords: presenilins interactome, Alzheimer's disease, pathological ageing

1. Introduction

Major clinical hallmarks of Alzheimer's disease (AD) are memory loss and cognitive impairment. Pathologically, AD is manifested by overproduction of toxic intracellular β-amyloid (Aβ) oligomers, deposited into extracellular senile plaques (SPs), and by hyperphosphorylation of tau protein deposited into neurofibrillary tangles (NFTs). Aβ is processed by the γ-secretase complex, where the most important component is presenilin [1]. There are two major types of AD: early-onset AD (EOAD), often linked with familial AD (FAD), and late-onset AD (LOAD), linked with sporadic AD (SAD). Familial EOAD represents 5–10% of all cases of AD and is associated with mutations in *PSEN1* encoding presenilin (PS1), *PSEN2* encoding presenilin 2 (PS2), and *APP* encoding amyloid β protein precursor (APP) [2, 3]. Overall, presenilins and APP mutations directly cause a production of toxic assemblies of oligomerized Aβ, followed by a formation of senile plaques [4]. Toxic Aβ forms induce apoptosis, oxidative stress, unfolded protein stress response, inflammation, or disturbances in calcium signalling, of which many are present in pathological ageing or in Alzheimer's disease.

Normal ageing results from natural maturational processes, whereas pathological ageing is related to non-normative factors such as disease or trauma to the brain. Ageing disproportionately affects frontal lobes [5]. Substantial overlap between ageing and neurodegeneration was demonstrated in several brain autopsy studies of aged people with no record of neurological diseases. These reports showed the presence of amyloid plaques, neurofibrillary tangles, Lewy bodies, inclusions of TAR DNA-binding protein 43 (TDP-43), synaptic dystrophy, and loss of neurons in most of ageing brains [6, 7]. However, unlike AD, pathological ageing usually lacks cognitive impairment despite similar senile plaque [8]. It was found that oxidative stress, commonly accompanying both ageing and AD, causes pathogenic conformational change of PS1 in neurons in vitro, which was followed by an increased ratio of Aβ42/40. It was further concluded that this conformational shift and deregulation of PS1 precedes Aβ deposition in pathological ageing [9]. These data demonstrated a direct connection between presenilins and PA. Presenilins contribute to brain pathology not only by deposition of toxic Aβ. Both PS1 and PS2 have been found to be involved in the regulation of apoptosis in neurons induced by trophic withdrawal or Aβ and via Jun Kinase pathway, respectively [10]. What is more, the role of presenilins in the progression of AD and PA is underlined by their numerous functions in the adult cerebral cortex functions, including maintenance of synaptic plasticity, long-term memory, and neuronal survival, which are critical for normal ageing, healthy brain, and cognitive ability [11].

Summarizing, presenilin functions can be controlled at different cellular levels, that is, (1) gene architecture, together with the influence of damaging genetic variants, in *PSEN1* and *PSEN2*, (2) gene expression, together with corresponding regulatory protein networks, (3) protein structure with its enzymatic activity, controlled by the assembly of the γ-secretase complex with accompanying partners and by post-translational modifications (phosphorylation and ubiquitination), (4) quantity, quality and availability of numerous substrates of presenilins and finally (5) by the interaction with molecular partners involved in numerous biological processes. Hereby, we highlighted that presenilins can determine different physiological and pathological processes by the interplay with diverse signal transduction pathways and by processing of various substrates. Generally, presenilins form a signalling network, which is critical for both AD and PA. Therefore, we present below molecular players that might affect biological functions of presenilins forming together so-called presenilin interactome.

2. Presenilin genetic structure and transcriptional regulation network

Presenilins 1 and 2 are encoded by homologous genes *PSEN1* and *PSEN2*, located at chromosomes 14q24.3 and 1q42.1, respectively [12, 13]. The genomic sizes of *PSEN1* and *PSEN2* are largely different, and it is 70 kb for *PSEN1* and 24 kb for *PSEN2*. *PSEN1* contains 13 exons and three first exons are located in the 5′ untranslated region (5′UTR) [14]. The first two exons and exon 9 of *PSEN1* could be alternatively spliced, causing structural changes to the protein [15]. *PSEN2* contains 12 exons and two first are located in the 5′ UTR [16]. The alternatively spliced products in *PSEN2* include in-frame omissions of exon 8 and simultaneous omissions of exons 3 and 4 [17]. Moreover, it has been found that splicing of exon 5 in *PSEN2* occurred under hypoxic stress conditions [18]. The transcription of *PSEN1* depends on two promoters producing two mRNA transcripts of 2.7 and 7.5 kb, with different 5′ UTRs [15]. *PSEN2* is also transcribed into two different transcripts of 2.4 and 2.8 kb [16].

Transcriptional regulation of presenilins might have an implication in AD and PA pathogenesis. Promoters of *PSENs* lack a TATA box but contain transcriptionally active GC. *PSEN1* promoter contains GC boxes corresponding to Sp1-like transcriptional factor, and the most active region is located between −22 and −6 bp. Transcriptional co-activator p300 with histone acetyl-transferase (HAT) activates *PSEN1* transcription. In particular in neuronal system, enhanced transcription of *PSEN1* was observed upon stimulation by N-methyl-D-aspartate (NMDA) or brain-derived neurotrophic factor (BDNF), under control of cAMP-responsive element binding (CREB). *PSEN1* expression and risk of AD and premature PA are also influenced by *PSEN1* promoter polymorphisms, found at −22C/T and −48C/T positions. Another suppressor of presenilin 1 is p53 protein that recruits other proteins to occupy *PSEN1* promoter [19]. Relatively little is known on the transcriptional regulation of *PSEN2*, where the promoter is located in a CpG island and is regulated by early growth response gene-1 (Egr-1) transcription factor, involved in learning and memory processes [20]. In addition, *PSEN2* promoter has been found to be regulated by nerve growth factor (NGF), with an NGF-responsive element localized between −403 and +13 [19]. Interestingly, parkin protein, known to be associated with Parkinson's disease, was found to act as a transcriptional factor modulating trans-activation of *PSEN1* and *PSEN2* promoters via RING1-IBR-RING2 domain and to influence γ-secretase activity [21]. The expression of both *PSEN1* and *PSEN2* was also described to be under thigh control of inflammatory cytokines, including tumour necrosis factor (TNF)-α, interferon (IFN)-γ, interleukin (IL)-1 β, IL-10 or TGF-β1 [22]. Generally, transcriptional regulation of presenilins is based on the complex signalling cascades controlling promoter's activation and requires a large variety of transcriptional factors. The dense network of signalling pathways related to the regulation of the promoters of *PSEN1* and *PSEN2* indicates numerous cellular processes that may contribute to the incidence and progression of AD and PA.

3. Presenilin structure and expression patterns

Structurally, PS1 and PS2 are integral membrane proteins of 467 and 448 amino acids, respectively [14, 15]. The homology between PS1 and PS2 is about 67%, with the highest similarity in transmembrane domains (TMDs). PS1 and PS2 comprise nine TM, among them TM1-6 are located at N′-terminal and TM7-9 at the C′-terminal. The catalytic centre with aspartate residues is located at the cytoplasmic side of TM6 and TM7, forming large hydrophilic loop (HL) [14]. Presenilins are activated by endoproteolysis yielding N′-terminal and C′-terminal portions. Endoproteolytical cleavage of PS1 occurs at HL, with the predominant cleavage site between amino acids 291 and 292, generating 28 kDa N′-terminal and 17 kDa C′-terminal fragments [23]. Similarly, PS2 is endoproteolytically cleaved into 35 kDa N′-terminal and 20 kDa C′-terminal fragment [24]. The most common mutations of presenilins occur in gene portion encoding C′-terminal, containing proline, alanine and leucin residues, and are usually loss of function for presenilins [25]. Due to protein structure complexity, presenilins interact with different partners, which will be *described in detail in Section 6*.

Presenilins are ubiquitously expressed, with some tissue-specific differences. Generally, *PSEN1* transcript is expressed at higher levels than *PSEN2*. The expression pattern of *PSEN1* and *PSEN2* in the brain is similar and present in different brain cells, such as cortical neurons, hippocampal neurons, granule cells or neurons of amygdala [26], and different types of glial cells [27]. In neurons, presenilins are expressed in the cell body and dendrites [28] and are localized in several subcellular compartments, that is, rough endoplasmic reticulum, Golgi complex, mitochondria, and at plasma membrane [29]. Moreover, presenilins were found to be expressed in several non-nervous cells and tissues, including lymphoblasts, fibroblasts, liver, spleen, and kidney [15].

4. Presenilin biological functions

Presenilins are aspartyl proteases and constitute a subunit of γ-secretase complex involved in the processing of APP and producing various Aβ peptides (*described in Section 5*). Besides that, presenilins are involved in numerous biological processes, playing various molecular functions in distinct subcellular compartments. Presenilins reprocess more than 90 substrates [30]. Presenilin substrates are involved in various signalling pathways, and several examples are provided in subsequent text.

Receptor tyrosine-protein kinase erbB-4 (ErbB4) processing by presenilins leads to enhanced spine formation through activation of Rac signalling [31]. Furthermore, presenilin-dependent cleavage of ErbB4 interplay is crucial for signal transduction during cells maturation [32]. Importantly, ErbB4 is involved in EGF/neuregulin signalling crucial for cell proliferation, differentiation, apoptosis, oligodendrocyte maturation, angiogenesis, synapse formation, LTP, and nerves myelination [33]. Another presenilin substrate of great biological importance is E-cadherin, which misprocessing affects transcriptionally regulated genes downstream of E-cadherin, involved in cell adhesion [34]. Next to that, glutamate receptor proteolysis performed by γ-secretase complex was found to be crucial for synaptic transmission [35]. Furthermore, VEGF receptor proteolysis and phosphorylation controlled by presenilins were reported to be important for angiogenesis, what could have further consequences in damages of brain areas by interfering with oxygen and energy supply [36]. Presenilin substrates selection is also a way of modulation of cell signalling and processing of presenilins' substrates regulated by the γ-secretase substrate-recruiting factors (γSSRFs) [37]. This establishes a complex signalling network of the process important in brain, thus in PA and AD.

Summarizing, presenilin biological functions and resultant interactome are not merely attributed to the γ-secretase activity and APP processing. Diversity of presenilin substrates is reflected by numerous biological implications including postsynaptic Ca^{2+} signalling, synaptogenesis, neurites outgrowth, lipid metabolism, cell adhesion, axon guidance, cell growth, regulation of dendritic spines, angiogenesis, LTP or glutamate synaptic transmission [30 (Tables 1 and 2), 38, 39]. In this regard, the amyloid cascade is complemented with the above-listed processes disturbed in AD. Similarly, pathological ageing is manifested by a loss of protein homeostasis, DNA damage, lysosomal dysfunction, epigenetic changes, immune deregulation, or disturbed calcium homeostasis [6]. Altogether, AD and PA might result from presenilin-dependent processes or presenilins' interactomes.

5. Presenilin substrate APP and production of toxic β-amyloid peptides

Aβ peptides are generated from amyloid β-precursor protein (APP) by enzymatic digestion involving the activity of α-, β- and γ-secretases. Amyloidogenic cleavage of APP is started by β-secretase, which generates a 100-kDa-soluble N-terminal fragment and membrane-bound 12-kDa C-terminal fragment (C99), which is further cleaved by γ-secretase, yielding the APP intracellular domain (AICD) and 40, 42, up to 56 amino acids Aβ peptides. C99 cleavage by γ-secretase is inaccurate and results in numerous different Aβ species, but those ending at position 40 (Aβ1-40) are the most abundant and considered as physiological (~80–90%), followed by less abundant but toxic 42 (Aβ1–42, ~5–10%). The second cleavage, which takes place within the hydrophobic transmembrane domain (TMD) and is regulated by intramembrane proteolysis (RIP), has been attributed to the γ-secretase complex with presenilins, as the catalytic component. The γ-secretase is a membrane-bound protease complex consisting of four components: nicastrin, anterior pharynx-defective 1 (APH-1) and presenilin enhancer 2 (PEN-2) and presenilin (1 or 2) forming aspartyl protease subunit and activity centre of the complex [40, 41].

As mentioned above, PA patients are characterized by the presence of amyloid deposits. However, PA is manifested by fewer-cored plaques and there is little or no neuritic pathology or neurofibrillary tangles in the cortex. Moreover, the species of Aβ peptides in PA differs from AD brains. It has been demonstrated that Aβ1–40 levels were 20-fold higher in AD brains compared to PA brains, whereas Aβ1–42 levels were only twofold higher [42]. Overall, several studies suggested quantitative and qualitative differences in the amyloid deposits between PA and AD brains [43]. It can be concluded that a wide spectrum of harmful effects of Aβ species, peptides, oligomers or plaques coincides with the disturbed presenilin signalling. These data demonstrate both common and different mechanisms of AD and PA, with the contribution presenilin, whose functions influence qualitative and quantitative status of amyloid.

6. Presenilin interactome: implementation in AD and PA

Numerous studies have been conducted in order to identify proteins interacting with PS1 and PS2. Majority of these studies have focused on the key signalling cascades specific for AD, as well as for PA, that is, oxidative stress, generation of free radicals or inflammatory processes. The best studied presenilin partners are components of γ-secretase complex (nicastrin, APH-1 and PEN-2), presenilin substrates (APP, Notch) and proteins involved in a regulation of cell death, calcium homeostasis and cell adhesion. It should be stressed that the knowledge on full PS interactome is crucial for more detailed definition of the pathomechanisms of AD and PA, and further studies are needed to complement this image.

6.1. The γ-secretase complex partners

Direct partners of presenilins are the components of the γ-secretase complex, namely nicastrin, APH-1 and PEN-2 [44]. Nicastrin associates with the complex comprising PS1-C′ terminal and APH-1 [45]. Nicastrin is required for the assembly of presenilin complexes to mediate Notch signalling and for processing and trafficking of β-amyloid precursor protein and thus plays a role in amyloid plaque formation [46]. Proper signalling between presenilin and nicastrin is important not only for processing of APP and accumulation of Aβ peptides but also for synaptic plasticity [47]. The next component of γ-secretase complex is PEN-2, a membrane protein with two predicted transmembrane domains, both N′ and C′ terminals are in extracellular space and with hydrophilic cytosolic loop [48]. PEN-2 binds to the fourth transmembrane domain of PS and helps to stabilize the γ-secretase complex after PS endoproteolysis [49]. Together with APH-1, PEN-2 is indispensable for Notch signalling [50], exhibiting thus similar properties like nicastrin. Importantly, mutations in TM4 reduced PS1-PEN-2 interaction which was further accompanied by an increased Aβ42 production and disrupted the endoplasmic reticulum calcium homeostasis [51]. The final component of γ-secretase complex is APH-1, a protein composed of seven transmembranes with N-terminus and large loops at cytosolic side [52]. APH-1 contains a conserved GXXXG motif that may be involved in interactions with other subunits of the complex [53]. APH-1 together with nicastrin forms a stable complex that constitutes a scaffold prior to the generation of the full presenilin complex [54]. APH-1 directly interacts with both immature and mature forms of the presenilins and nicastrin and this is indispensable for γ-secretase activity [55]. According to that described above, presenilin biological functions are regulated by complex assembly.

6.2. Mitochondrial interactome of presenilins

The γ-secretase complex was found in mitochondria [56]. Since Aβ is not a substrate for mitochondrial γ-secretase complex, its mitochondrial implication may be related to cell death signalling, switching between necrosis and apoptosis depending on ATP levels [56]. Moreover, PS2 was found to modulate ER-mitochondria juxtaposition and interactions, and that was enhanced in the case of PS2 mutations [57]. In detail, the components of γ-secretase complex were found in mitochondria-associated ER membranes (MAMs) with lipid raft-like domain [58]. Mutations in presenilin 1 were found to impair the IP3 receptor- and voltage-dependent calcium transport, as well as Ca^{2+}-dependent mitochondrial proteins transport, and this was followed by a mitochondrial dysfunction, reduced patients' motor coordination and Aβ aggregation with ultimate dementia [59]. Presenilin 1 was found to interact with mitochondrial intramembrane cleaving protease, called presenilin-associated rhomboid-like protein (PARL), which could promote changes in mitochondrial morphology [60]. Next to mitochondrial membrane residing proteins, presenilins interact with immunophilin FKBP38 forming macromolecular complexes, which promoted anti-apoptotic protein Bcl-2 sequestration into endoplasmic reticulum and Golgi apparatus compartments [61]. Importantly, AD-linked presenilin mutants enhanced the pro-apoptotic activity by reducing levels of mitochondrial Bcl-2 [62]. In the light of above, presenilins and other elements of the γ-secretase complex located in mitochondria establish a novel type of cellular signalling and interacting network.

6.3. Hif-1α interaction

Hypoxia-inducible factor 1α (Hif-1α), which upregulates γ-secretase activity, was recently identified as PSs partner [63]. Hif-1α is related to ubiquitin-mediated proteolysis, induction of angiogenesis, inflammation or increase of vascular tone. Villa et al. [63] showed that Hif-1α acts as a subunit of γ-secretase activity, which is distinct from its canonical role as a transcription factor. Moreover, hypoxia-induced cell invasion and metastasis were improved by either γ-secretase inhibitors or a dominant-negative Notch coactivator, indicating essential role of γ-secretase/Notch signalling [63]. These data provided the molecular mechanism for an increased incidence of AD and PA following cerebral ischaemic injuries and strokes [64]. In addition, cells lacking presenilin 1 were characterized by an impaired induction of HIF-1α in response to hypoxia. Furthermore, presenilin 1 and HIF-1α physical interaction may protect HIF-1α from degradation through proteasome. Additionally, M146V Psen1 mutation impaired metabolic induction of HIF-1α [65]. These data suggest that PS1 regulates the induction of HIF-1α.

6.4. Presenilin interactome of tetraspanin-enriched microdomains (TEMs)

Tetraspanin-enriched microdomains (TEMs) consist of proteins and lipids crucial for coordination of many biological processes, including cell adhesion, proteolysis, cell motility or sorting to exosomes [66]. A series of proteins transiently interacting with the γ-secretase complex were found in TEM network. Moreover, the disruption of TEM inhibited Aβ production [67]. The study of Wakabayashi and co-workers showed an interaction of γ-secretase complex with tetraspanin proteins, that is, CD81, Upk1b and CD9 and cell surface immunoglobulin superfamily proteins EWI-2 and EWI-F [67]. Another research evidenced that the association of TEM with γ-secretase complex is needed for an enhancement of its proteolytic activity [68]. These data also confirmed a localization of γ-secretase in the raft-like domains [69]. All the above studies revealed that the integrity of tetraspanin microdomains is crucial for presenilins and γ-secretase signalling. In addition to TEM, presenilin complex and its interactive network were shown to be located predominantly in a specialized sub-compartment of ER, spatially and biochemically connected to mitochondria, called mitochondria-associated ER membranes (MAMs). MAM is a lipid raft-like structure, enriched in anionic phospholipids, cholesterol and sphingomyelin. MAM is involved in cholesterol and phospholipid metabolism, calcium homeostasis and in mitochondrial function and dynamics. MAM function was altered and ER–mitochondrial connectivity is significantly increased in AD. The authors of these findings proposed the "MAM-AD hypothesis" with a central role of ER–mitochondrial-presenilin network in AD pathogenesis [70]. Schon and Area-Gomez [71] reported a large list of genes encoded in MAM, including genes involved in the regulation of apoptosis process, maintenance of calcium signalling, inflammatory response (formation of inflammasomes) or protein ubiquitination. In addition, they discovered that a MAM function in cholesteryl ester and phospholipid synthesis was overactive in AD. According to Schon and Area-Gomez [71], MAM is an unexplored research area, and its importance is vastly underestimated in brain pathology, both AD and PA.

6.5. Recent findings on presenilin interactome

The large list of molecular partners of presenilins supports their extended significance in AD and PA. Testing whole presenilin interactome, instead of selected signalling pathway, is highly recommended due to the fact that any brain pathologies are extremely complex diseases, where causative and susceptibility genes are highly interconnected [72]. Novel PSEN-related genes were discovered through high-throughput immunoaffinity (co-IP and pull-down) studies [73, 74]. Novel findings on PS1 partners involved ST13, GCDH, ECSIT and CDC37 proteins, and novel PS2 partners were PDCD4, DYNC1H1 and ECSIT. These interactions together with the already known might provide a novel and holistic insight into the molecular pathways interconnection underlying various brain pathologies. Soler-López and co-workers also indicated and confirmed a physical connection between apolipoprotein E (APOE) and PS1 [73, 74]. Direct evidence on APOE and PS1 binding provided a novel insight into the pathogenic role of APOE as a regulator of PS1 in APP cleavage. Furthermore, Soler-López et al. also confirmed an interaction between PS1 and PS2, previously suggested to cooperate as part of the γ-secretase complex in APP cleavage [73, 74]. The direct binding of APP with both PS1 and PS2, confirmed by co-IP, had been previously suggested [75]. These results provided a fresh perspective on the possible functions of presenilin in the process of brain degeneration in AD or PA.

Furthermore, the interaction of presenilin with ECSIT components (evolutionarily conserved signalling intermediates in Toll pathway) could constitute a molecular link between oxidative stress, inflammation and mitochondrial dysfunction in AD. Supporting the idea of the implication of presenilins' interactome in oxidative stress response, another component of redox signalling, glutaryl-CoA dehydrogenase (GCDH), also interacts with PS. Moreover, the association of ECSIT with APOE was shown to bind Aβ in its oxidized form Ref. [76]. Another novel example of presenilin interaction partners is the member of the tumour necrosis factor receptor-associated factor (TRAF) family. More precisely, presenilin full-length holo-proteins were suggested to be novel substrates of TRAF6-mediated Lysine-63-linked ubiquitination. Furthermore, TRAF6 induced PS1 gene transcription in a JNK-dependent manner. Notably, TRAF6-mediated ubiquitination of presenilin did not affect γ-secretase enzyme activity, but likely regulated presenilin function in calcium signalling. TRAF6 deficiency coincided with reduced PS1 ubiquitination, protein levels and Ca^{2+} leakage from ER, suggesting that ubiquitination may be an important regulatory post-translational modification of presenilin function [77]. On the other hand, TRAF6 is involved in nerve growth factor (NGF)-dependent phosphorylation, ubiquitination and association of tropomyosin receptor kinase A (TrkA) with p75NTR, thereby promoting cell survival and differentiation. Under pathological conditions in AD or PA, pro-NGF stimulation can lead to nitrosylation of TrkA, thereby impairing its ubiquitination and downstream signalling which results in apoptosis [78]. In addition, presenilin ubiquitination was shown to be controlled by ubiquilin 1. In detail, ubiquilin 1 promoted the formation of PS1-positive aggregosomes [79, 80]. Furthermore, PS1 ubiquitination was found to demand Cdc4 component of the SCF ubiquitin E2-E3 ligase complex (Skp1-Cdc53/CUL1-F-box protein) and formation of this complex was followed by an increase in Aβ production [81]. Overall, the above-described scientific reports present a large spectrum and different aspects of presenilin interactome, important for brain functions thus implemented in brain pathological ageing or degeneration.

6.6. Presenilins and synaptic transmission

One of the most important pathologies of brain degeneration or pathological ageing is disturbed synaptic transmission. It is believed that the impairment of synaptic function accounts for pathological ageing or degeneration independently on SP deposition. Recently, presenilins were proposed to participate in neurotransmitter release in the γ-secretase function-independent manner. It was reported that presenilins are essential for regulating neurotransmitter release like glutamate, and its inhibition is mediated by a depletion of ER Ca^{2+} storage and a block of intracellular Ca^{2+} release [82]. Importantly, PS1 knockout and PS1-M146V neurons did not exhibit synaptic strengths. On the other hand, synaptic activity was found to modulate PS1 activity and Aβ40/42 ratio via altering PS1 conformation [83]. Additionally, it has recently been demonstrated that the interaction of PS1 with synaptic vesicle-associated protein, synaptotagmin 1 (Syt1), implicated novel synaptic functions of PS1, and both proteins modulated each other's functions in neurons via direct activity-triggered interaction, and the PS1-Syt1 complexes were crucial for exocytosis at the synapses and safeguarding of PS1 conformation [84]. Overall, mounting evidence points to a role of presenilins in synaptic transmission. It is clear that the interplay between presenilins and synaptic activity could originate from presenilins γ-secretase activity.

6.7. Other aspects of interactomes of presenilins 1 and 2

PS1 and PS2 can exhibit distinct from γ-secretase activities [85]. For instance, it has been demonstrated that autophagy and lysosomal proteolysis required presenilin 1 [86], as well as presenilin 2 through a γ-secretase-independent mechanism [87]. Further detailed analyses revealed novel interactions of the γ-secretase core complex with a molecular machinery targeting synaptic vesicles to cellular membranes, and with the H^+-transporting lysosomal ATPase macrocomplex [88]. Importantly, lysosomal dysfunction is also associated with many age-related pathologies like Parkinson's and Alzheimer's disease, as well as with a decline in lifespan. Conversely, targeting lysosomal functional capacity is emerging as a means to promote longevity [89]. Another example of γ-secretase-independent interaction is the catenin/

cadherin network that was almost exclusively found associated with PS1. In detail, catenin $\alpha2$, catenin $\beta1$ and plakophilin 4, as well as the cadherins 2 and 11, were repeatedly and strongly enriched in the PS1-specific sample [90]. On the other hand, an intramembrane protease, signal peptide peptidase (SPP), predominantly co-purified with PS2-containing γ-secretase complexes and was observed to influence Aβ production [90]. Another interesting interaction was found between PS2 and DREAM protein [91]. The Ca^{2+}-binding protein DREAM regulates gene transcription and activity of potassium channels in neurons. DREAM interaction with PS2 might have implication in the regulation of the Ca^{2+} content in endoplasmic reticulum. The transient co-expression of DREAM and presenilin 2 potentiated the decrease of endoplasmic reticulum Ca^{2+} observed in presenilin-overexpressing cells. This could be due to a direct effect of DREAM on presenilin 2 as the two proteins interacted in a Ca^{2+}-independent fashion. Finally, an example of an interaction unique to PS2 is the DRAL protein. DRAL is an LIM-only protein containing four LIM domains and an N-terminal half LIM domain. The PS2-DRAL interaction was confirmed using yeast two-hybrid and immunoaffinity studies, suggesting that DRAL functioned as an adaptor protein that links PS2 to an intracellular signalling [92]. This paragraph outlines the differences between PS1 and PS2, and cautions against correct attributing of a given interactome with disease phenotype.

7. Pathological ageing and Alzheimer's disease in the *omic* era

The above-presented insight on the presenilins' interactome provides important information about the background of pathological ageing and neurodegeneration. Nevertheless, the protein interactome is still only a small fragment recognized by the systemic biology. Thus, there is a need to integrate interactome data with other high-throughput data. The importance of integration of different parts of biological systems is stressed by the fact of becoming an ageing society. Undoubtedly, the ageing is one of the major risk factors for various diseases, ranging from cancer, cardiovascular diseases, type 2 diabetes (T2D) and ending with Alzheimer's disease. This creates a long list of ageing-related diseases (ARDs). In this regard, a recognition of the whole functional network linking ageing and ARD becomes one of the key tasks of current medical science. In the era of *omics* research, publicly available domains allow comparison of genomics, transcriptomics, proteomics, metabolomics, miRomics, epigenomics, regulomics (regulatory genomics), microbiomics, and lipidomics with particular diseasome [93]. These criteria are met by the 'GeroNet' research model, an approach that is targeting the relationship between ageing and hundreds of ARD [94]. These studies indicated several subnetworks associated with ageing, including 'response to reduced oxygen levels' or 'cell cycle checkpoints'. Importantly, the GeroNet model has helped to identify several genes that may play a key role combining pathological ageing and Alzheimer's disease, including the top five most significant STAT3, P53, FOS, BCL2 and NFKB1. The next example of integration of several omics research is analysis of the genes associated with longevity and ageing, collected in Ageing Gene/Interventions database (http://www.kaeberleinlab.org/ageid) and in GenAge database, which can be useful for the research on different interactome networks in AD or PA. Another recent *omic* approach was presented in the studies on inflammaging with propagation of pro- and anti-inflammatory mediators in a dynamic manner from cell to cell and from organ to organ, supplemented by glycomics data [95]. Additionally, other wide-genomic studies revealed longevity and age-related functional biological networks, underlining the importance of neuronal development, autophagy and other processes associated with Alzheimer's diseases [96]. Furthermore, the integration of various systemic biology data has revealed common mechanisms associated with genomic instability and reduced capacity to DNA repair for both ageing and neurodegeneration. [97, 98]. Genomic instability is also influenced by a number of epigenetic changes that can be associated with both ageing and AD. These epigenetic changes occur at different levels, for example, histone methylation pattern, replacement of the canonical histones by rare variants of histones or regulated by an altered expression of non-coding RNA [99]. Indeed, there are studies confirming a decrease in genome-wide DNA methylation occurring in both ageing and AD patients [100]. Significantly, epigenetic regulation of the presenilins 1 and 2 was found to be pivotal in the development of the cerebral cortex of mice [101]. This epigenetic regulation of PS1 and PS2 was controlled by the acetylation and methylation of histone H3K9/14 and this was associated with further differential expression of PS1 and PS2, as well as their interacting protein partners. These data indicated that multiple levels of epigenetic regulation may be involved in controlling the formation of amyloid beta. Given epigenetic context, interestingly, dietary supplementation with B group vitamins restored methylation of promoters of presenilin 1, APP and BACE1 and slowed down the progression of AD [102]. In addition, this was associated with a decrease in oxidative stress and a delay in the accumulation of neurological symptoms in transgenic mice with beta amyloid pathology [102]. Generally, the methylation status of all the elements of presenilins' interactome may be suitable for future research on ageing and AD. Supplementing the above data, an important matter in the era of omics research is the use of appropriate computational and mathematical models. One example is weighted gene co-expression network analysis method (WGCNA), which by the use of large omics data may predict gene-gene, protein-protein, or gene-miRNA interaction nature [103]. In particular, the WGCNA method was used to organize gene expression data into a functionally significant structure, in order to indicate the modules of co-expressed genes and novel gene signatures associated with Alzheimer's disease [104].

Overall, ADs or PAs are systemic diseases based on the interplay of several cellular networks. Thus, it should be noted that conducting the research only on individual protein factors, as the studies on presenilins and processing of APP, is only a part of the holistic homeostatic insight on these pathological states and such comprehensive approach is still missing in the discussion. Due to wide-range nature of ageing and degeneration process, the conducted studies should be more non-deterministic, without a concrete causation and particular trigger (gene, protein pathway). The holistic approach should include the response to DNA repair with cell cycle and genome integrity checkpoints, proteostasis, unfolded protein response, protein-folding chaperone networks, ER-associated degradation/ubiquitin proteasome system, endo-lysosomal network, autophagy, inflammatory response and other stress-response networks. This can be accomplished by integration of various omics data and can be fulfilled when supported by latest methods and research approaches including next-generation sequencing, modern neuroimaging or high-throughput computational bioinformatic studies. Complexity and multi-level nature of the network of genes, proteins, their interactomes and relationships with ageing-related disease processes present in both AD and PA have been reported in several recent review papers [94, 98, 105–107]. This and other reviews underline the importance of the integration of different biological data provided for the process of brain degeneration, in both PA and AD, and other neurodegeneration disorders with dementia.

8. Challenges of the future

The aim of the future will be to develop an accurate map of omic data of the ageing process. This is associated with the problem of collection of the samples for multiomics data from a human across lifespan. Second, the factors that can be a source of a noise in the omic data should be identified, including information on the ethnicity, personal immunological history or parameters of lifestyle (dietary habits, physical activity and microbiological status). Comprehensive of integrative interactomics of (epi)gene-protein-pathways axis would demand more advanced and consolidated computational, mathematical and bioinformatic tools. These methods should integrate the data obtained with a use of various methodological approaches and engines, from different biological range and integrate the statistical power for all of them. Further aspects, which require to be consolidated or demand additional computational approaches, are related to the source material (tissues and cells) used for omics analyses. These and other criteria must be met to be able to pinpoint the cause and prevent a decline in cognitive skills, so important in everyone's life.

9. Summary

Neurodegeneration in AD or PA is a multiparametrical process. Thus, there is a need of not only for an establishment of the most complete genetic background but also to pinpoint the functional implications of this knowledge. Despite strong efforts of the recent research, based mostly on modern technologies, including GWAS and WES, it is still a largely unknown domain. It is very likely that expanding the interactomes PS1 and PS2 will help to emerge the complex biological processes accompanying processing of many substrates of presenilins. The broad spectrum of γ-secretase substrates and interacting proteins has invoked the analogy to γ-secretase 'secretosome' or 'proteasome of the membrane'. The complexity of the interactome of presenilin 1 is implicated in a number of molecular functions, manifested in different cell components and implicated in a variety of biological processes, crucial for Alzheimer's disease and pathological ageing, and is depicted in a schematic presentation of this chapter (**Figure 1**). Additionally, it is important to take into account environmental factors, for example, psychological circumstances might affect gene expression profile via epigenetical mechanisms, and thus presenilins interacting network, with further functional implications. In conclusion, the understanding of existing genetic mechanisms together with presenilin functions leading to brain degeneration in AD or PA is crucial for better understanding of molecular bases of these pathologies and facing them in the future.

http://dx.doi.org/10.5772/intechopen.68748

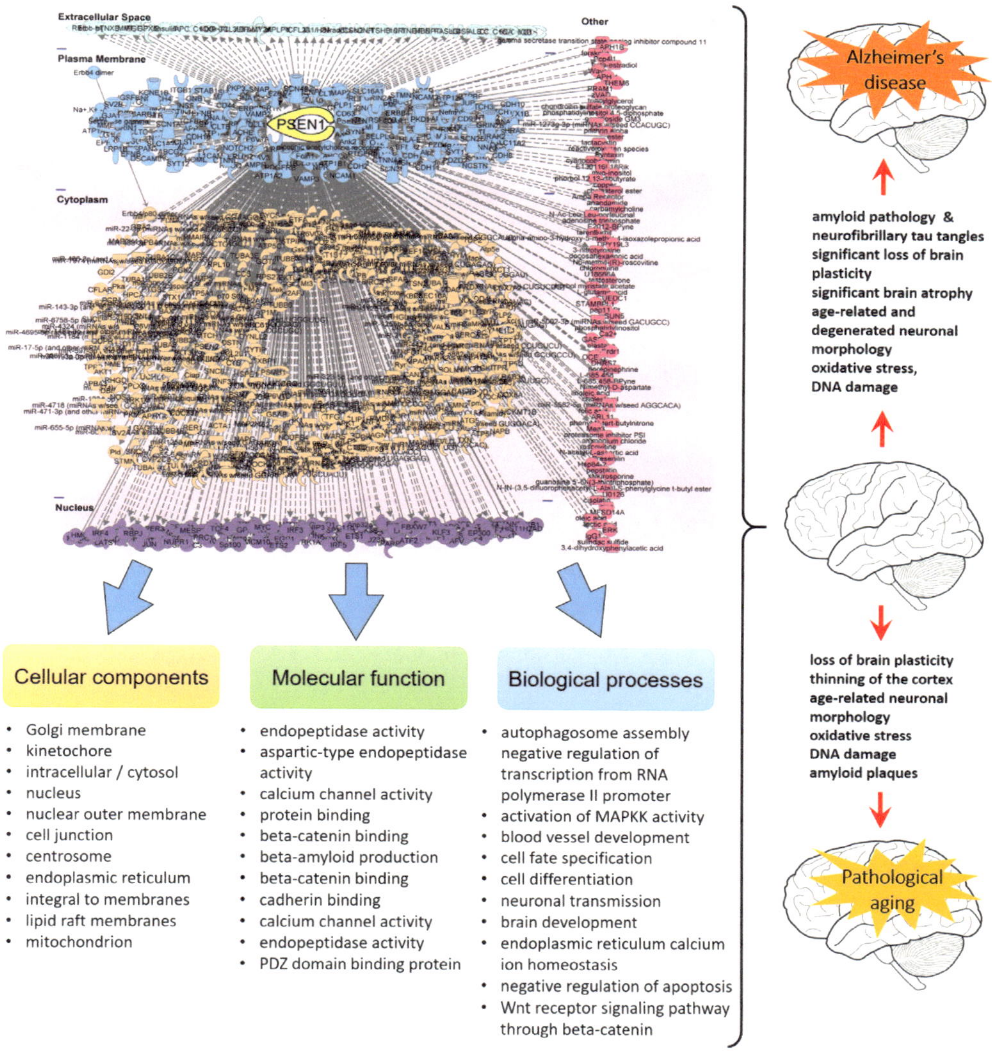

Figure 1. The interactome of presenilin 1 in Alzheimer's disease and in pathological ageing. Presenilin 1 interactome was generated using Ingenuity Pathway Analysis software (www.ingenuity.com). Presenilin 1 interactome is implicated in a number of molecular functions, cell components and biological processes of presenilin 1, according to GeneCards®: The Human Gene Database. Presenilin 1 interaction network with its functional consequences are crucial both for Alzheimer's disease and for pathological ageing brains.

Acknowledgements

This work was supported by the National Science Centre (Poland) grant 'SONATA6' no. G1119-2013/09/D/NZ3/01348 and by Statutory Grant of Mossakowki Medical Research Centre from Ministry of Science and Higher Education.

Author details

Michalina Maria Wężyk[1,2]* and Cezary Żekanowski[1]

*Address all correspondence to: mwezyk@imdik.pan.pl

1 Department of Neurodegenerative Disorders, Laboratory of Neurogenetics, Mossakowski Medical Research Centre Polish Academy of Sciences, Warsaw, Poland

2 Department of Neurology, Warsaw Medical University, Warsaw, Poland

References

[1] Serrano-Pozo A, Frosch MP, Masliah E, Hyman BT. Neuropathological alterations in Alzheimer disease. Cold Spring Harbor Perspectives in Medicine. 2011;**1**:a006189. DOI: 10.1101/cshperspect.a006189

[2] Cruts M, Theuns J, Van Broeckhoven C. Locus-specific mutation databases for neurodegenerative brain diseases. Human Mutations. 2012;**33**:1340-1344. DOI: 10.1002/humu.22117

[3] Zekanowski C, Styczyńska M, Pepłońska B, Gabryelewicz T, Religa D, Ilkowski J, Kijanowska-Haładyna B, Kotapka-Minc S, Mikkelsen S, Pfeffer A, Barczak A, Łuczywek E, Wasiak B, Chodakowska-Zebrowska M, Gustaw K, Łaczkowski J, Sobów T, Kuźnicki J, Barcikowska M. Mutations in presenilin 1, presenilin 2 and amyloid precursor protein genes in patients with early-onset Alzheimer's disease in Poland. Experimental Neurology. 2003;**184**:991-996. DOI: 10.1002/humu.22117

[4] Weggen S, Beher D. Molecular consequences of amyloid precursor protein and presenilin mutations causing autosomal-dominant Alzheimer's disease. Alzheimer's Research & Therapy. 2012;**30**:9. DOI: 10.1186/alzrt107

[5] Pfefferbaum A, Adalsteinsson E, Sullivan EV. Frontal circuitry degradation marks healthy adult aging: Evidence from diffusion tensor imaging. Neuroimage. 2005;**26**:891-899. DOI: 10.1186/alzrt107

[6] Wyss-Coray T. Ageing, neurodegeneration and brain rejuvenation. Nature. 2016;10;**539**: 180-186. DOI: 10.1038/nature20411

[7] Elobeid A, Libard S, Leino M, Popova SN, Alafuzoff I. Altered proteins in the aging brain. Journal of Neuropathology and Experimental Neurology. 2016;**75**:316-325. DOI: 10.1093/jnen/nlw002

[8] Murray ME, Dickson DW. Is pathological aging a successful resistance against amyloid-beta or preclinical Alzheimer's disease? Alzheimer's Research & Therapy. 2014;**6**:24. DOI: 10.1186/alzrt254. eCollection 2014

[9] Wahlster L, Arimon M, Nasser-Ghodsi N, Post KL, Serrano-Pozo A, Uemura K, Berezovska O. Presenilin-1 adopts pathogenic conformation in normal aging and in sporadic Alzheimer's disease. Acta Neuropathologica. 2013;**125**:187-199. DOI: 10.1007/s00401-012-1065-6

[10] Wolozin B, Maheshwari S, Jones C, Dukoff R, Wallace W, Racchi M, Nagula S, Shulman NR, Sunderland T, Bush A. Beta-amyloid augments platelet aggregation: Reduced activity of familial angiopathy-associated mutants. Molecular Psychiatry. 1998;**3**:500-507

[11] Wines-Samuelson M, Shen J. Presenilins in the developing, adult, and aging cerebral cortex. Neuroscientist. 2005;**11**:441-451

[12] Cruts M, Backhovens H, Wang SY, Van Gassen G, Theuns J, De Jonghe CD, Wehnert A, De Voecht J, De Winter G, Cras P, et al. Molecular genetic analysis of familial early-onset Alzheimer's disease linked to chromosome 14q24.3. Human Molecular Genetics. 1995;**4**:2363-2371

[13] Cruts M, Hendriks L, Van Broeckhoven C. The presenilin genes: A new gene family involved in Alzheimer disease pathology. Human Molecular Genetics. 1996;**5**:1449-1455

[14] Sherrington R, Rogaev EI, Liang Y, Rogaeva EA, Levesque G, Ikeda M, Chi H, Lin C, Li G, Holman K, Tsuda T, Mar L, Foncin JF, Bruni AC, Montesi MP, Sorbi S, Rainero I, Pinessi L, Nee L, Chumakov I, Pollen D, Brookes A, Sanseau P, Polinsky RJ, Wasco W, Da Silva HA, Haines JL, Perkicak-Vance MA, Tanzi RE, Roses AD, Fraser PE, Rommens JM, St George-Hyslop PH. Cloning of a gene bearing missense mutations in early-onset Alzheimer's disease. Nature. 1995;**29**:754-760

[15] Rogaev EI, Sherrington R, Wu C, Levesque G, Liang Y, Rogaeva EA, Ikeda M, Holman K, Lin C, Lukiw WJ, de Jong PJ, Fraser PE, Rommens JM, St George-Hyslop P. Analysis of the 5′ sequence, genomic structure, and alternative splicing of the presenilin-1 gene (PSEN1) associated with early onset Alzheimer disease. Genomics. 1997;**40**:415-424.

[16] Levy-Lahad E, Bird TD. Genetic factors in Alzheimer's disease: A review of recent advances. Annals in Neurology. 1996;**40**:829-840

[17] Prihar G, Fuldner RA, Perez-Tur J, Lincoln S, Duff K, Crook R, Hardy J, Philips CA, Venter C, Talbot C, Clark RF, Goate A, Li J, Potter H, Karran E, Roberts GW, Hutton M, Adams MD. Structure and alternative splicing of the presenilin-2 gene. Neuroreport. 1996;**7**:1680-1684

[18] Higashide S, Morikawa K, Okumura M, Kondo S, Ogata M, Murakami T, Yamashita A, Kanemoto S, Manabe T, Imaizumi K. Identification of regulatory cis-acting elements for alternative splicing of presenilin 2 exon 5 under hypoxic stress conditions. Journal of Neurochemistry. 2004;**91**:1191-1198

[19] Chen XF, Zhang YW, Xu H, Bu G. Transcriptional regulation and its misregulation in Alzheimer's disease. Molecular Brain. 2013;**21**:44. DOI: 10.1186/1756-6606-6-44.

[20] Ounallah-Saad H1, Beeri R, Goshen I, Yirmiya R, Renbaum P, Levy-Lahad E. Transcriptional regulation of the murine presenilin-2 gene reveals similarities and differences to its human orthologue. Gene. 2009;**446**:81-89. DOI: 10.1016/j.gene.2009.06.015

[21] Duplan E, Sevalle J, Viotti J, Goiran T, Bauer C, Renbaum P, Levy-Lahad E, Gautier CA, Corti O, Leroudier N, Checler F, da Costa CA. Parkin differently regulates presenilin-1 and presenilin-2 functions by direct control of their promoter transcription. Journal of Molecular & Cell Biology. 2013;**5**:132-142. DOI: 10.1093/jmcb/mjt003

[22] Saura CA. Presenilin/gamma-secretase and inflammation. Frontiers in Aging Neuroscience. 2010;**18**:16. DOI: 10.3389/fnagi.2010.00016.

[23] Podlisny MB, Citron M, Amarante P, Sherrington R, Xia W, Zhang J, Diehl T, Levesque G, Fraser P, Haass C, Koo EH, Seubert P, St George-Hyslop P, Teplow DB, Selkoe DJ. Presenilin proteins undergo heterogeneous endoproteolysis between Thr291 and Ala299 and occur as stable N- and C-terminal fragments in normal and Alzheimer brain tissue. Neurobiology Disease. 1997;**3**:325-337

[24] Tomita T, Maruyama K, Saido TC, Kume H, Shinozaki K, Tokuhiro S, Capell A, Walter J, Grünberg J, Haass C, Iwatsubo T, Obata K. The presenilin 2 mutation (N141I) linked to familial Alzheimer disease (Volga German families) increases the secretion of amyloid beta protein ending at the 42nd (or 43rd) residue. Proceedings of the National Academy of Sciences United States of America. 1997;**94**:2025-2030

[25] De Strooper B, Iwatsubo T, Wolfe MS. Presenilins and γ-secretase: Structure, function, and role in Alzheimer disease. Cold Spring Harbor Perspectives in Medicine. 2012;**2**: a006304. DOI: 10.1101/cshperspect.a006304.

[26] Lee MK, Slunt HH, Martin LJ, Thinakaran G, Kim G, Gandy SE, Seeger M, Koo E, Price DL, Sisodia SS. Expression of presenilin 1 and 2 (PS1 and PS2) in human and murine tissues. Journal of Neuroscience. 1996;**16**:7513-7525

[27] Miake H, Tsuchiya K, Nakamura A, Ikeda K, Levesque L, Fraser PE, St-George Hyslop PH, Mizusawa H, Uchihara T. Glial expression of presenilin epitopes in human brain with cerebral infarction and in astrocytoma. Acta Neuropathologica. 1999;**98**:337-340

[28] Cook DG, Sung JC, Golde TE, Felsenstein KM, Wojczyk BS, Tanzi RE, Trojanowski JQ, Lee VM, Doms RW. Expression and analysis of presenilin 1 in a human neuronal system: Localization in cell bodies and dendrites. Proceedings of the National Academy of Sciences United States of America. 1996;**93**:9223-9228

[29] Kovacs DM, Fausett HJ, Page KJ, Kim TW, Moir RD, Merriam DE, Hollister RD, Hallmark OG, Mancini R, Felsenstein KM, Hyman BT, Tanzi RE, Wasco W. Alzheimer-associated presenilins 1 and 2: Neuronal expression in brain and localization to intracellular membranes in mammalian cells. Nature Medicine. 1996;**2**:224-229

[30] Haapasalo A, Kovacs DM. The many substrates of presenilin/γ-secretase. Journal of Alzheimer's Disease. 2011;**25**:3-28. DOI: 10.3233/JAD-2011-101065

[31] Inoue E, Deguchi-Tawarada M, Togawa A, Matsui C, Arita K, Katahira-Tayama S, Sato T, Yamauchi E, Oda Y, Takai Y. Synaptic activity prompts gamma-secretase-mediated cleavage of EphA4 and dendritic spine formation. Journal of Cell Biology. 2009;**185**:551-564. DOI: 10.1083/jcb.200809151

[32] Hoeing K, Zscheppang K, Mujahid S, Murray S, Volpe MV, Dammann CE, Nielsen HC. Presenilin-1 processing of ErbB4 in fetal type II cells is necessary for control of fetal lung maturation. Biochimica et Biophysica Acta. 2011;**1813**:480-491. DOI: 10.1016/j.bbamcr.2010.12.017

[33] Vidal GA, Naresh A, Marrero L, Jones FE. Presenilin-dependent gamma-secretase processing regulates multiple ERBB4/HER4 activities. Journal of Biological Chemistry. 2005;**280**: 19777-19783

[34] Marambaud P, Shioi J, Serban G, Georgakopoulos A, Sarner S, Nagy V, Baki L, Wen P, Efthimiopoulos S, Shao Z, Wisniewski T, Robakis NK. A presenilin-1/gamma-secretase cleavage releases the E-cadherin intracellular domain and regulates disassembly of adherens junctions. EMBO Journal. 2002;**21**:1948-1956

[35] Meyer EL, Strutz N, Gahring LC, Rogers SW. Glutamate receptor subunit 3 is modified by site-specific limited proteolysis including cleavage by g-secretase. Journal of Biological Chemistry. 2003;**278**:23786-23796

[36] Cai J, Chen Z, Ruan Q, Han S, Liu L, Qi X, Boye SL, Hauswirth WW, Grant MB, Boulton ME. γ-Secretase and presenilin mediate cleavage and phosphorylation of vascular endothelial growth factor receptor-1. Journal of Biological Chemistry. 2011;**286**:42514-42523. DOI: 10.1074/jbc.M111.296590

[37] Barthet G, Georgakopoulos A, Robakis NK. Cellular mechanisms of γ-secretase substrate selection, processing and toxicity. Progress in Neurobiology. 2012;**98**:166-175. DOI: 10.1016/j.pneurobio.2012.05.006

[38] Armstrong RA. What causes Alzheimer's disease? Folia Neuropathologica. 2013;**51**: 169-188

[39] Crews L, Masliah E. Molecular mechanisms of neurodegeneration in Alzheimer's disease. Human Molecular Genetics. 2010;**19**:R12-R20. DOI: 10.1093/hmg/ddq160

[40] Zhang YW1, Thompson R, Zhang H, Xu H. APP processing in Alzheimer's disease. Molecular Brain. 2011;**4**:3. DOI: 10.1186/1756-6606-4-3

[41] Small DH, Klaver DW, Foa L. Presenilins and the gamma-secretase: Still a complex problem. Molecular Brain. 2010;**3**:7. DOI: 10.1186/1756-6606-3-7

[42] Moore BD, Chakrabarty P, Levites Y, Kukar TL, Baine AM, Moroni T, Ladd TB, Das P, Dickson DW, Golde TE. Overlapping profiles of Aβ peptides in the Alzheimer's disease and pathological aging brains. Alzheimer's Research & Therapy. 2012;**4**:18. DOI: 10.1186/alzrt121

[43] Maarouf CL, Daugs ID, Kokjohn TA, Walker DG, Hunter JM, Kruchowsky JC, Woltjer R, Kaye J, Castaño EM, Sabbagh MN, Beach TG, Roher AE. Alzheimer's disease and non-demented high pathology control nonagenarians: Comparing and contrasting the biochemistry of cognitively successful aging. PLoS One. 2011;**6**:e27291. DOI: 10.1371/journal.pone.0027291

[44] Verdile G, Gandy SE, Martins RN. The role of presenilin and its interacting proteins in the biogenesis of Alzheimer's beta amyloid. Neurochemical Research. 2007;**32**:609-623

[45] Bergman A, Laudon H, Winblad B, Lundkvist J, Näslund J. The extreme C terminus of presenilin 1 is essential for gamma-secretase complex assembly and activity. Journal of Biological Chemistry. 2004;**279**:45564-45572

[46] Sesele K, Thanopoulou K, Paouri E, Tsefou E, Klinakis A, Georgopoulos S. Conditional inactivation of nicastrin restricts amyloid deposition in an Alzheimer's disease mouse model. Aging Cell. 2013;**12**:1032-1040. DOI: 10.1111/acel.12131

[47] Lee L, Dale E, Staniszewski A, Zhang H, Saeed F, Sakurai M, Fa' M, Orozco I, Michelassi F, Akpan N, Lehrer H, Arancio O. Regulation of synaptic plasticity and cognition by SUMO in normal physiology and Alzheimer's disease. Scientific Reports. 2014;**4**:7190. DOI: 10.1038/srep07190

[48] Crystal AS, Morais VA, Pierson TC, Pijak DS, Carlin D, Lee VM, Doms RW. Membrane topology of gamma-secretase component PEN-2. Journal of Biological Chemistry. 2003;**278**:20117-20123

[49] Watanabe N, Tomita T, Sato C, Kitamura T, Morohashi Y, Iwatsubo T. Pen-2 is incorporated into the gamma-secretase complex through binding to transmembrane domain 4 of presenilin 1. Journal of Biological Chemistry. 2005;**280**:41967-41975

[50] Francis R, McGrath G, Zhang J, Ruddy DA, Sym M, Apfeld J, Nicoll M, Maxwell M, Hai B, Ellis MC, Parks AL, Xu W, Li J, Gurney M, Myers RL, Himes CS, Hiebsch R, Ruble C, Nye JS, Curtis D. aph-1 and pen-2 are required for Notch pathway signaling, gamma-secretase cleavage of betaAPP, and presenilin protein accumulation. Developmental Cell. 2002;**3**:85-97

[51] Chen WT, Hsieh YF, Huang YJ, Lin CC, Lin YT, Liu YC, Lien CC, Cheng IH. G206D mutation of presenilin-1 reduces Pen2 interaction, increases Aβ42/Aβ40 ratio and elevates ER Ca(2+) accumulation. Molecular Neurobiology. 2015;**52**:1835-1849. DOI: 10.1007/s12035-014-8969-1

[52] Fortna RR, Crystal AS, Morais VA, Pijak DS, Lee VM, Doms RW. Membrane topology and nicastrin-enhanced endoproteolysis of APH-1, a component of the gamma-secretase complex. Journal of Biological Chemistry. 2004;**279**:3685-3693

[53] Lee SF, Shah S, Yu C, Wigley WC, Li H, Lim M, Pedersen K, Han W, Thomas P, Lundkvist J, Hao YH, Yu G. A conserved GXXXG motif in APH-1 is critical for assembly and activity of the gamma-secretase complex. Journal of Biological Chemistry. 2004;279:4144-4152

[54] Lee SF, Shah S, Li H, Yu C, Han W, Yu G. Mammalian APH-1 interacts with presenilin and nicastrin and is required for intramembrane proteolysis of amyloid-beta precursor protein and Notch. Journal of Biological Chemistry. 2002;277:45013-45019

[55] Gu Y, Chen F, Sanjo N, Kawarai T, Hasegawa H, Duthie M, Li W, Ruan X, Luthra A, Mount HT, Tandon A, Fraser PE, St George-Hyslop P. APH-1 interacts with mature and immature forms of presenilins and nicastrin and may play a role in maturation of presenilin.nicastrin complexes. Journal of Biological Chemistry. 2003;**278**:7374-7380

[56] Hansson CA, Frykman S, Farmery MR, Tjernberg LO, Nilsberth C, Pursglove SE, Ito A, Winblad B, Cowburn RF, Thyberg J, Ankarcrona M. Nicastrin, presenilin, APH-1, and PEN-2 form active gamma-secretase complexes in mitochondria. Journal of Biological Chemistry. 2004;**279**:51654-51660

[57] Zampese E, Fasolato C, Pozzan T, Pizzo P. Presenilin-2 modulation of ER-mitochondria interactions: FAD mutations, mechanisms and pathological consequences. Communicative & Integrative Biology. 2011;**4**:357-360. DOI: 10.4161/cib.4.3.15160

[58] Area-Gomez E, Del Carmen Lara Castillo M, Tambini MD, Guardia-Laguarta C, de Groof AJ, Madra M, Ikenouchi J, Umeda M, Bird TD, Sturley SL, Schon EA. Upregulated function of mitochondria-associated ER membranes in Alzheimer disease. EMBO Journal. 2012;**31**:4106-4123. DOI: 10.1038/emboj.2012.202

[59] Sepulveda-Falla D, Barrera-Ocampo A, Hagel C, Korwitz A, Vinueza-Veloz MF, Zhou K, Schonewille M, Zhou H, Velazquez-Perez L, Rodriguez-Labrada R, Villegas A, Ferrer I, Lopera F, Langer T, De Zeeuw CI, Glatzel M. Familial Alzheimer's disease-associated presenilin-1 alters cerebellar activity and calcium homeostasis. Journal of Clinical Investigation. 2014;**124**:1552-1567. DOI: 10.1172/JCI66407

[60] Hill RB, Pellegrini L. The PARL family of mitochondrial rhomboid proteases. Seminar in Cell Developmental Biology. 2010;**21**:582-592. DOI: 10.1016/j.semcdb.2016.07.034

[61] van de Hoef DL, Bonner JM, Boulianne GL. FKBP14 is an essential gene that regulates presenilin protein levels and Notch signaling in Drosophila. Development. 2013;**140**:810-819. DOI: 10.1242/dev.081356

[62] Wang HQ, Nakaya Y, Du Z, Yamane T, Shirane M, Kudo T, Takeda M, Takebayashi K, Noda Y, Nakayama KI, Nishimura M. Interaction of presenilins with FKBP38 promotes apoptosis by reducing mitochondrial Bcl-2. Human Molecular Genetics. 2005;**14**: 1889-1902

[63] Villa JC, Chiu D, Brandes AH, Escorcia FE, Villa CH, Maguire WF, Hu CJ, de Stanchina E, Simon MC, Sisodia SS, Scheinberg DA, Li YM. Nontranscriptional role of Hif-1α in activation of γ-secretase and notch signaling in breast cancer. Cell Reproduction. 2014;**8**: 1077-1092

[64] Zhang X, Zhou K, Wang R, Cui J, Lipton SA, Liao FF, Xu H, Zhang YW. Hypoxia-inducible factor 1alpha (HIF-1alpha)-mediated hypoxia increases BACE1 expression and beta-amyloid generation. Journal of Biological Chemistry. 2007;**282**:10873-10880

[65] De Gasperi R, Sosa MA, Dracheva S, Elder GA. Presenilin-1 regulates induction of hypoxia inducible factor-1α: altered activation by a mutation associated with familial Alzheimer's disease. Molecular Neurodegeneration. 2010;**5**:38. DOI: 10.1186/1750-1326-5-38

[66] Seipold L, Saftig P. The emerging role of tetraspanins in the proteolytic processing of the amyloid precursor protein. Frontiers in Molecular Neuroscience. 2016;**9**:149. DOI: 10.3389/fnmol.2016.00149

[67] Wakabayashi T, Craessaerts K, Bammens L, Bentahir M, Borgions F, Herdewijn P, Staes A, Timmerman E, Vandekerckhove J, Rubinstein E, Boucheix C, Gevaert K, De Strooper B. Analysis of the gamma-secretase interactome and validation of its association with tetraspanin-enriched microdomains. Nature Cell Biology. 2009;**1-1**:1340-1346. DOI: 10.1038/ncb1978

[68] Perez-Hernandez D, Gutiérrez-Vázquez C, Jorge I, López-Martín S, Ursa A, Sánchez-Madrid F, Vázquez J, Yáñez-Mó M. The intracellular interactome of tetraspanin-enriched microdomains reveals their function as sorting machineries toward exosomes. Journal of Biological Chemistry. 2013;**288**:11649-11661. DOI: 10.1074/jbc.M112.445304

[69] Hattori C, Asai M, Onishi H, Sasagawa N, Hashimoto Y, Saido TC, Maruyama K, Mizutani S, Ishiura S. BACE1 interacts with lipid raft proteins. Journal of Neuroscience Research. 2006;**84**:912-917.

[70] Area-Gomez E, Schon EA. Mitochondria-associated ER membranes and Alzheimer disease. Current Opinion in Genetic Development. 2016;**38**:90-96. DOI: 10.1016/j.gde. 2016.04.006

[71] Schon EA, Area-Gomez E. Mitochondria-associated ER membranes in Alzheimer disease. Molecular & Cell Neuroscience. 2013;**55**:26-36. DOI: 10.1016/j.mcn.2012.07.011

[72] Oti M, Brunner HG. The modular nature of genetic diseases. Clinical Genetics. 2007;**71**:1-11

[73] Soler-López M, Badiola N, Zanzoni A, Aloy P. Towards Alzheimer's root cause: ECSIT as an integrating hub between oxidative stress, inflammation and mitochondrial dysfunction. Hypothetical role of the adapter protein ECSIT in familial and sporadic Alzheimer's disease pathogenesis. Bioessays. 2012;**34**:532-541. DOI: 10.1002/bies.201100193

[74] Soler-López M, Zanzoni A, Lluís R, Stelzl U, Aloy P. Interactome mapping suggests new mechanistic details underlying Alzheimer's disease. Genome – Research. 2011;**21**:364-376. DOI: 10.1101/gr.114280.110

[75] Xia W, Zhang J, Perez R, Koo EH, Selkoe DJ. Interaction between amyloid precursor protein and presenilins in mammalian cells: Implications for the pathogenesis of Alzheimer disease. Proceedings of the National Academy of Science United States of America. 1997;94:8208-8213

[76] Strittmatter WJ, Weisgraber KH, Huang DY, Dong LM, Salvesen GS, Pericak-Vance M, Schmechel D, Saunders AM, Goldgaber D, Roses AD. Binding of human apolipoprotein E to synthetic amyloid beta peptide: Isoform-specific effects and implications for late-onset Alzheimer disease. Proceedings of the National Academy of Science United States of America. 1993;90:8098-8102

[77] Yan R, Farrelly S, McCarthy JV. Presenilins are novel substrates for TRAF6-mediated ubiquitination. Cell Signal. 2013;**25**:1769-1779. DOI: 10.1016/j.cellsig.2013.05.015

[78] Zheng C, Geetha T, Gearing M, Babu JR. Amyloid β-abrogated TrkA ubiquitination in PC12 cells analogous to Alzheimer's disease. Journal of Neurochemistry. 2015;**133**:919-925. DOI: 10.1111/jnc.13076

[79] Thomas AV, Herl L, Spoelgen R, Hiltunen M, Jones PB, Tanzi RE, Hyman BT, Berezovska O. Interaction between presenilin 1 and ubiquilin 1 as detected by fluorescence lifetime imaging microscopy and a high-throughput fluorescent plate reader. Journal of Biological Chemistry. 2006;**281**:26400-26407

[80] Viswanathan J, Haapasalo A, Böttcher C, Miettinen R, Kurkinen KM, Lu A, Thomas A, Maynard CJ, Romano D, Hyman BT, Berezovska O, Bertram L, Soininen H, Dantuma NP, Tanzi RE, Hiltunen M. Alzheimer's disease-associated ubiquilin-1 regulates presenilin-1 accumulation and aggresome formation. Traffic. 2011;**12**:330-348. DOI: 10.1111/j.1600-0854.2010.01149.x

[81] Li J, Pauley AM, Myers RL, Shuang R, Brashler JR, Yan R, Buhl AE, Ruble C, Gurney ME. SEL-10 interacts with presenilin 1, facilitates its ubiquitination, and alters A-beta peptide production. Journal of Neurochemistry. 2002;**82**:1540-1548

[82] Zhang C, Wu B, Beglopoulos V, Wines-Samuelson M, Zhang D, Dragatsis I, Südhof TC, Shen J. Presenilins are essential for regulating neurotransmitter release. Nature. 2009;**460**:632-636. DOI: 10.1038/nature08177

[83] Dolev I, Fogel H, Milshtein H, Berdichevsky Y, Lipstein N, Brose N, Gazit N, Slutsky I. Spike bursts increase amyloid-β 40/42 ratio by inducing a presenilin-1 conformational change. Nature Neuroscience. 2013;**16**:587-595. DOI: 10.1038/nn.3376. PubMed PMID: 23563578

[84] oltowska KM, Maesako M, Lushnikova I, Takeda S, Keller LJ, Skibo G, Hyman BT, Berezovska O. Dynamic presenilin 1 and synaptotagmin 1 interaction modulates exocytosis and amyloid β production. Molecular Neurodegeneration. 2017;**12**:15. DOI: 10.1186/s13024-017-0159-y

[85] Lai MT, Chen E, Crouthamel MC, DiMuzio-Mower J, Xu M, Huang Q, Price E, Register RB, Shi XP, Donoviel DB, Bernstein A, Hazuda D, Gardell SJ, Li YM. Presenilin-1 and presenilin-2 exhibit distinct yet overlapping gamma-secretase activities. Journal of Biological Chemistry. 2003;**278**:22475-22481

[86] Zhang X, Garbett K, Veeraraghavalu K, Wilburn B, Gilmore R, Mirnics K, Sisodia SS. A role for presenilins in autophagy revisited: Normal acidification of lysosomes in cells lacking PSEN1 and PSEN2. Journal of Neuroscience. 2012;**32**:8633-8648. DOI: 10.1523/JNEUROSCI.0556-12.2012

[87] Neely KM, Green KN. Presenilins mediate efficient proteolysis via the autophagosome-lysosome system. Autophagy. 2011;**7**:664-665

[88] Wolfe DM, Lee JH, Kumar A, Lee S, Orenstein SJ, Nixon RA. Autophagy failure in Alzheimer's disease and the role of defective lysosomal acidification. European Journal of Neuroscience. 2013;**37**:1949-1961. DOI: 10.1111/ejn.12169

[89] Carmona-Gutierrez D, Hughes AL, Madeo F, Ruckenstuhl C. The crucial impact of lysosomes in aging and longevity. Ageing Research Review. 2016;**32**:2-12. DOI: 10.1016/j.arr.2016.04.009

[90] Jeon AH, Böhm C, Chen F, Huo H, Ruan X, Ren CH, Ho K, Qamar S, Mathews PM, Fraser PE, Mount HT, St George-Hyslop P, Schmitt-Ulms G. Interactome analyses of mature γ-secretase complexes reveal distinct molecular environments of presenilin (PS) paralogs and preferential binding of signal peptide peptidase to PS2. Journal of Biological Chemistry. 2013;**288**:15352-15366. DOI: 10.1074/jbc.M112.441840

[91] Fedrizzi L, Lim D, Carafoli E, Brini M. Interplay of the Ca^{2+}-binding protein DREAM with presenilin in neuronal Ca^{2+} signaling. Journal of Biological Chemistry. 2008;**283**: 27494-27503. DOI: 10.1074/jbc.M804152200

[92] Tanahashi H, Tabira T. Alzheimer's disease-associated presenilin 2 interacts with DRAL, an LIM-domain protein. Human Molecular Genetics. 2000;**9**:2281-2289

[93] Wysocki K, Ritter L. Diseasome: An approach to understanding gene-disease interactions. Annual Review in Nursing Research. 2011;**29**:55-72

[94] Yang J, Huang T, Song WM, Petralia F, Mobbs CV, Zhang B, Zhao Y, Schadt EE, Zhu J, Tu Z. Discover the network mechanisms underlying the connections between aging and age-related diseases. Scientific Reports. 2016;**6**:32566. DOI: 10.1038/srep32566

[95] Monti D, Ostan R, Borelli V, Castellani G, Franceschi C. Inflammaging and human longevity in the omics era. Mechanisms of Ageing and Development. 2016 Dec 27. pii: S0047-6374(16)30261-5. DOI: 10.1016/j.mad.2016.12.008. [Epub ahead of print]

[96] Walter S, Atzmon G, Demerath EW, Garcia ME, Kaplan RC, Kumari M, Lunetta KL, Milaneschi Y, Tanaka T, Tranah GJ, Völker U, Yu L, Arnold A, Benjamin EJ, Biffar R, Buchman AS, Boerwinkle E, Couper D, De Jager PL, Evans DA, Harris TB, Hoffmann W, Hofman A, Karasik D, Kiel DP, Kocher T, Kuningas M, Launer LJ, Lohman KK, Lutsey PL, Mackenbach J, Marciante K, Psaty BM, Reiman EM, Rotter JI, Seshadri S, Shardell MD, Smith AV, van Duijn C, Walston J, Zillikens MC, Bandinelli S, Baumeister SE, Bennett DA, Ferrucci L, Gudnason V, Kivimaki M, Liu Y, Murabito JM, Newman AB, Tiemeier H, Franceschini N. A genome-wide association study of aging. Neurobiological Aging. 2011;**32**:2109.e15-e28. DOI: 10.1016/j.neurobiolaging.2011.05.026

[97] Chow HM, Herrup K. Genomic integrity and the ageing brain. Nature Review Neuroscience. 2015;**16**:672-684. DOI: 10.1038/nrn4020

[98] Maslov AY, Vijg J. Genome instability, cancer and aging. Biochimica et Biophysica Acta. 2009;**1790**:963-969. DOI: 10.1016/j.bbagen.2009.03.020

[99] Mastroeni D, Grover A, Delvaux E, Whiteside C, Coleman PD, Rogers J. Epigenetic mechanisms in Alzheimer's disease. Neurobiological Aging. 2011;**32**:1161-1180. DOI: 10.1016/j.neurobiolaging.2010.08.017

[100] Kumar A, Thakur MK. Epigenetic regulation of presenilin 1 and 2 in the cerebral cortex of mice during development. Developmental Neurobiology. 2015;**75**:1165-1173. DOI: 10.1002/dneu.22274

[101] Pal S, Tyler JK. Epigenetics and aging. Science Advances. 2016;**2**:e1600584. DOI: 10.1126/sciadv.1600584

[102] Fuso A, Nicolia V, Cavallaro RA, Ricceri L, D'Anselmi F, Coluccia P, Calamandrei G, Scarpa S. B-vitamin deprivation induces hyperhomocysteinemia and brain S-adenosylhomocysteine, depletes brain S-adenosylmethionine, and enhances PS1 and BACE expression and amyloid-beta deposition in mice. Molecular & Cell Neuroscience. 2008;**37**:731-746. DOI: 10.1016/j.mcn.2007.12.018

[103] Langfelder P, Horvath S. WGCNA: An R package for weighted correlation network analysis. BMC Bioinformatics. 2008;**9**:559. DOI: 10.1186/1471-2105-9-559

[104] Miller JA, Oldham MC, Geschwind DH. A systems level analysis of transcriptional changes in Alzheimer's disease and normal aging. Journal of Neuroscience. 2008;**28**: 1410-1420. DOI: 10.1523/JNEUROSCI.4098-07.2008

[105] Smita S, Lange F, Wolkenhauer O, Köhling R. Deciphering hallmark processes of aging from interaction networks. Biochimica et Biophysica Acta. 2016;**1860**:2706-2715. DOI: 10.1016/j.bbagen.2016.07.017

[106] Castrillo JI, Oliver SG. Alzheimer's as a systems-level disease involving the interplay of multiple cellular networks. Methods in Molecular Biology. 2016;**1303**:3-48. DOI: 10.1007/978-1-4939-2627-5_1

[107] Nahálková J. The protein-interaction network with functional roles in tumorigenesis, neurodegeneration, and aging. Molecular & Cell Biochemistry. 2016;**423**:187-196

Chapter 7

Is Senescence Important in Hepatic Diseases?

Ruth Pacheco Rivera, Jaime Arellanes Robledo and
Jesús Serrano Luna

Additional information is available at the end of the chapter

http://dx.doi.org/10.5772/intechopen.68587

Abstract

Aging is a condition in which a person gradually loses the ability to maintain homeostasis, due to structural alteration or dysfunction. Aging changes biological processes in many organs and tissues. The loss of regenerative capacity is the most dramatic age-associated alteration in the liver. Cellular damage, if not repaired, leads to apoptosis or senescence. The presence of permanent cell cycle arrest, the acquisition of major morphological change, and expression of senescence-associated β-galactosidase (SA-β-gal) are the characteristics of cellular senescence (CS). Interestingly, CS plays a crucial role in aging of both individual organs and the entire organism; consequently, senescent cells accumulate in organs and decline in organ function. Senescent cells have considerable influence on their microenvironment and exert both beneficial and detrimental effects through secretory associated senescent phenotype (SASP) factors. CS has attracted considerable recent interest with recognition of pathways linking aging, malignancy, and insulin resistance and the current focus on therapeutic interventions to extend healthspan. There are major implications for hepatology in the field of fibrosis and cancer, where cellular senescence of hepatocytes, cholangiocytes, stellate cells, and immune cells has been implicated in chronic liver disease progression.

Keywords: senescence, aging, chronic liver diseases

1. Introduction

Aging is a biological process that consists of a series of structural and functional changes that appear over time and are not a consequence of diseases or accidents. In general, tissues are comprised of specific cells that determine the tissue microenvironment. Various factors affect the cellular environment, such as oxygen pressure, oxidative stress, temperature, and several growth factors secreted by cells. Sometimes the cell's microenvironment alters the tissue homeostasis, causing a permissive environment that favors tumor promotion and development. This progressive aging is caused by multiple factors. The following nine characteristics are generally considered to contribute to the aging process: altered intracellular communication, genomic instability, telomere attrition, epigenetic alterations, loss of proteostasis, deregulated nutrient sensing, mitochondrial dysfunction, stem cells exhaustion, and cellular senescence [1].

2. Cellular senescence

Cellular senescence (CS) is a stable form of cell cycle arrest that limits the proliferative potential of cells [2]. Senescence is the result of various degenerative changes characterized by shortening of the telomeres, chromosomic instability, DNA damage, oxidative stress producing reactive oxygen species (ROS), and oncogene overexpression [3–10]. Some researchers consider CS the natural solution to prevent cell damage, which may lead to various diseases including cancer. In contrast, with age, CS is considered to promote several chronic diseases. The pathological effects of CS may affect the health of elderly people due to the accumulation of senescent cells in several organs and tissues because CS can impair tissue regeneration. Furthermore, senescent cells can release several molecules, such as growth factors, cytokines, and chemokines that alter cellular homeostasis [11].

Up to date, two basic mechanisms have been identified to induce senescence: replicative senescence and premature senescence. Replicative senescence, or the Hayflick limit, is associated with telomere attrition; telomere exhaustion causes the limited proliferative capacity of certain types of *in vitro* cultured cells [12]. Cells react to the loss of telomeres as if it is DNA damage, which therefore triggers the DNA damage response (DDR); the cellular response is similar to that initiated by external agents, for example, ionizing radiation and drugs.

In contrast, premature senescence is related to chromosomic instability, DNA damage, oxidative stress, oncogene overexpression, and epigenetic changes. Senescent cells have a typical morphology in culture: cells are enlarged, vacuolated, and flattened and in some cases, they are multinucleated. However, *in vivo* senescent cells retain the normal morphology according to the tissue to which they belong. It has been found that these cells are metabolically active, and they can secrete growth factors, chemokines, and metalloproteases; this is known as the senescence associated secretor phenotype (SASP) [13].

2.1. Senescence markers

Senescent cells have several typical characteristics. First, they are positive for β-galactosidase activity at a suboptimal pH (pH 6), and this activity is based on the increment of lysosomal activity. One limitation of the β-gal assay is the need to use fresh or frozen samples [14]. Another characteristic is that senescent cells are in cellular arrest. Cellular arrest is an essential condition for senescence to occur, as senescent cells are positive for Ki67 protein or negative for the incorporation of 5-bromodeoxyuridine (Brdu) [15]. Other senescent markers are related to tumor suppressors such as p53, p16, p21, and the hypophosphorylated Rb protein. Heterochromatin bodies are known as heterochromatin foci in the nucleolus. In cells with DNA damage, it is common to find γ-H2AX histone phosphorylation which carries the DDR. Another finding is the decrease in lamin B1 levels as a common feature in many types of senescence [16, 17]. On the other hand, senescent cells have been found in biological processes other than aging as in systems such as humans, mice, and chicken embryos, suggesting that these cells are important to embryogenesis [18].

2.2. Senescence pathways

In the senescence process, there are two key tumor suppressors, the INK4/ARF locus and p53. The INK4/ARF locus allows the expression of three important proteins, $p16^{Ink4a}$, $p14^{Arf}$ ($p19^{Arf}$ in mice), and $p15^{Ink4b}$. Serrano et al. discovered the protein p16Ink4a. The $p16^{Ink4a}$ binds to CDK4/6 cyclins, preventing the phosphorylation of the Rb protein family; therefore, the cell cycle is inhibited at the G1 phase and cells enter in a cellular arrest, and this pathway is known as $p16^{Ink4a}$-Rb [19]. In contrast, p53 is a transcription factor, which transcribes target genes to regulate various biological cell processes in response to stress stimuli; the biological cell processes include apoptosis, senescence, energy metabolism, and antioxidant defense. p53 is stabilized and phosphorylated by upstream kinases including ataxia telangiectasia (ATM) and Chk2 [10, 20, 21]. Phosphorylated p53 upregulates the transcription of its target gene, p21, which activates the Rb protein through the inhibition of cyclin E/Cdk2. The hypophosphorylated Rb protein inhibits the transcription of E2F genes, including cyclin A and proliferating cell nuclear antigen (PCNA), which are required for cell cycle progression [22]. On the other hand, $p14^{Arf}$ is directly related to p53 and is linked to the mourin double murine 2 (Mdm2) protein; therefore, p53 is stabilized, and p21 is expressed and inhibits cyclin E/Cdk2 [23]. This senescent pathway is called the p53-p21 pathway. Another senescence-signaling pathway is through the p38 protein, which is a mitogen activated protein kinase (MAPK) protein that transforms a variety of stress stimuli into a common senescence signal [24]. The inactivation of p38 delays the onset of various forms of cellular senescence including replicative, oxidative-stress-induced, and oncogene induced senescence. In contrast, enforced activation of p38 by a constitutive active form MAPK kinase (MKK6EE) of upstream kinase, MKK6, acutely induces cellular senescence [25, 26].

In recent years, other elements have been incorporated into the senescence pathway regulation. Studies on genetic regulation in human fibroblasts and mice embryonic fibroblasts (MEFs) showed the presence of long noncoding RNAs (lncRNAs), which are derived from noncoding RNAs (ncRNAs). Tumor suppressors have specific lncRNAs; for example, several IncRNAs, such as focally amplified lncRNA on chromosome 1 (FAL 1), BRAF-activated non-protein coding RNA (BANCR), and long intervening noncoding RNAs (LINCRNA) p21, have been found in p21 [27–30]. In the case of p53, lncRNA metastasis associated lung adenocarcinoma transcript 1 (MALAT1) as well as 7SL have been related to p53 expression [31, 32]. The INK4a-ARF locus and p16INK4amRNA are linked with lncRNAs VAD, antisense non-coding RNA in the INK4 locus (ANRIL), MIR31 host gene (MIR31), and Urothelial cancer associated 1 (UCA 1) [33–38]. Another lncRNA associated with senescence is senescence-associated long non-coding RNA (SALNR), which is related to NF-9 [39]. telomeric repeat containing RNA (TERRA) is a lncRNA associated with telomere length [40]. Researchers have shown that lncRNAs are tightly regulated and tissue specific. Moreover, the dysregulation of lncRNAs has been associated with human diseases. Further studies must be performed to accurately determine the functional role of these lncRNAs in senescence and aging [41].

2.3. Chromatin alterations

Alterations in the structure of chromatin are believed to contribute to the irreversible nature of the senescent state. Narita et al. found that in DNA cells stained with 4',6-diamidino-2-phenylindole (DAPI), chromatin bodies called foci can be observed at the nucleus [42]. It is likely that DAPI-stained foci correspond to highly compacted heterochromatin, as senescent cell chromatin is resistant to micrococcal nuclease digestion; moreover, DAPI foci contain numerous proteins characteristic of transcriptionally inactive heterochromatin, including hypoacetylated histones, methylated histone H3 on Lys 9 (H3K9 me), and heterochromatin protein 1 (HP1). The formation of heterochromatin structures known as heterochromatin foci is associated with senescence-associated heterochromatin foci (SAHF). Various forms of stress induce SAHF formation as well as other senescence phenotypes, suggesting that SAHFs can be used to identify senescent cells *in vivo* and that SAHF formation somehow contributes to the mechanisms of cellular senescence; although, not all senescent cells exhibit SAHFs [43].

2.4. Oxidative stress and liver senescence

Under normal physiological conditions, cells are protected from oxidative stress by an array of endogenous antioxidants that maintain a balance between pro-oxidant production and antioxidant capacity. An imbalance occurs when intracellular antioxidants are unable to neutralize the pro-oxidants such as ROS, which are a number of highly reactive molecules derived from molecular oxygen [44]. ROS are mainly produced by the mitochondrial respiratory chain, cytochrome P450, and autooxidation of endogenous substrates such as heme proteins, catecholamines, quinones, among others [45]. ROS exert a broad array of biological effects, ranging from physiological regulatory functions to several oxidative modifications, which can contribute to the pathogenesis of various diseases. ROS can also impact the cell by altering physiological and biochemical processes such as gene expression, cell adhesion, cell metabolism, cell cycle, cell disease, and cell death [46, 47]. Thus, oxidative stress has been confirmed to be a common participant in several diseases including liver diseases [48]. It has been proposed that the damage induced by oxidative stress may represent a common link between different chronic liver diseases. This proposal is supported by the fact that free radicals are key players not only in normal liver function but also in the genesis and progression of liver steatosis, fibrosis, cirrhosis, and hepatocellular carcinoma (HCC) [49, 50]. Therefore, a strong association is expected between oxidative stress and the pathogenesis of liver diseases. Oxidative stress is an inherent component in the liver as the activity of many enzymes involved in lipogenesis, fatty acid oxidation, cholesterol, and phospholipid metabolism is regulated by the redox status of liver parenchyma, which can influence the redox balance of the cell microenvironment [51]. Thus, following liver injury by different etiological factors [52], endogenously produced ROS may have an accumulative impact (mainly evidenced as an increase in lipid peroxidation), which plays a critical role in the progression of chronic liver diseases [53].

Several studies have proposed that ROS production is one of the main activators and stabilizers of CS. Although this is a preliminary proposal, there is evidence demonstrating a direct contribution of ROS to both the DDR and the redox-activated pathways [54, 55] and induces telomere shortening [56], which results in a DDR and senescence activation. Up to date, both experimental and clinical studies have strongly supported the association of CS with chronic liver diseases. In addition to specific parenchymal or nonparenchymal liver structures, studies have highlighted the appearance of CS in two paradoxical settings, as a tumor suppressor and as a tumor promoter, and in two physiological processes, aging and tissue repair [57, 58]. Cellular senescence is involved in multiple physiological processes; the complexity of CS may be elucidated by deciphering the mechanisms that induce its activation, such as oxidative stress. In this regard, evidence has shown that increased ROS production by mitochondrial dysfunction is triggered after a DDR and subsequent CS activation, which in turn is a consequence of p21 activation. The sequence of events maintains a dynamic feedback loop that is necessary for the stability of growth arrest during the establishment of the senescent phenotype [59]. A similar phenomenon was observed during the activation of the p16/RB pathway, which induces high intracellular levels of ROS and thereby activates protein kinase C-Δ (PKCΔ); consequently, further ROS are generated to establish a positive feedback loop to sustain ROS-PKCΔ signaling [60]. Other studies have reported that activation of the RAS, p21, and p53 pathways are also closely related to elevated ROS production [61, 62]. In these reports, N-acetylcysteine treatment blocked cell cycle arrest and thereby CS, demonstrating that ROS accumulation is an important mediator of CS; furthermore, researchers proposed that ROS are a causal agent of CS. The evidence confirms that ROS play a key role in the CS process; however, it is still unclear whether ROS are a consequence or cause of CS.

2.5. Reactive oxygen species and hepatic diseases

A variety of free radicals are found in the liver and can be classified as mitochondrial, principally from complexes I and III, and extra mitochondrial, such as cytochrome P450, xanthine oxidase, nitric oxide synthase, and nicotinamide adenine dinucleotide phosphate reduced (NADPH) oxidase. Where neutrophils and Kupffer cells primarily produce free radicals, the cytochrome P450 system and mitochondria are the major sites of ROS release in hepatocytes. An important mechanistic source of ROS is lipid metabolism, which is dependent on the redox balance of the liver, and its alteration is closely linked to both alcoholic and nonalcoholic steatohepatitis [51, 63]. The above-mentioned sources of ROS are strictly controlled in normal hepatocytes; however, in hepatic diseases, an overproduction of free radicals can overcome the antioxidant defenses and induce liver injury [51]. Consequently, the liver is a continuous target of oxidative stress and redox balance. It is not surprising that an increasing number of findings have shown a close association between liver diseases and ROS production [63]. Clinical and experimental reports have suggested that CS onset may be an intrinsic phenomenon from the beginning of liver injury, such as the appearance of neoplastic nodules [64, 65]. This proposal is supported by the presence of replicative and premature senescence in both parenchymal and nonparenchymal liver cells [58, 66, 67]. Using a liver injury model to mimic sequential HCC progression (from fibrosis to cirrhosis and HCC) [68], we recently confirmed that CS appearance is intrinsic to the initiation of liver injury, as a chronological increase of CS alongside HCC progression was observed [69]. We did not determine ROS levels in this investigation; however, HCC was induced with continuous diethylnitrosamine administration, a hepatotoxic and potent

ROS producer [70], suggesting that the chronological appearance of CS was accompanied by persistent ROS induction. In a recent study, the role of hepatocyte senescence in the development of insulin resistance was investigated [71]. Using HepG2 cells, they demonstrated that H_2O_2 treatment induced CS despite insulin stimulation. This phenomenon was accompanied by a persistent nuclear localization of FoxO1, a transcription factor that, among others, promotes the expression of genes involved in cell cycle arrest and detoxification of ROS. Moreover, an increase and decrease in the expression of glucose transporters 2 and 4 (GLUT2 and GLUT4), respectively, were proposed as senescence markers, as this pattern was found in senescent HepG2, in human cirrhotic liver tissue, and in publicly available liver disease datasets. In a different study by the same research group, gene expression profiles of HepG2 cells subjected to oxidative stress were compared with public microarray datasets obtained from human cirrhotic samples. The results showed that the gene upregulation profile of senescent HepG2 cells induced by H_2O_2 treatment was similar to that in human cirrhotic livers. Interestingly, gene expression profile patterns of senescent hepatocytes were markedly linked to alterations in cell cycle regulation, morphology, metabolism, and stellate cell activation, which occur alongside impaired synthetic function in senescence [72]. Although these results suggest a close relationship between hepatocyte senescence and ROS action, the use of an external stressor agent to induce CS may be a key factor to work in an asynchronous manner in the sequence of molecular events involved in intrinsic ROS production. More direct evidence has demonstrated a strong interconnection between senescence, ROS, and TGF-β signaling in chronic liver diseases. Borkham-Kamphorst et al. showed that the overexpression of cysteine-rich protein 61 (CCN1/CYR61) significantly inhibited the production of collagen type I and induced ROS, leading to CS and apoptosis *in vivo* and *in vitro*. This effect was associated with an attenuation of TGF-β signaling; as a result, CCN1/CYR61 overexpression mitigated liver fibrogenesis in a bile duct ligation model. This analysis is a clear example of ROS and CS induction as a potential molecular mechanism for tissue repair and remodeling promoted by the manipulation of CCN1/CYR61 during hepatic injury [73]. In a similar study with contrasting reports, dioscin, a saponin plant steroid, promoted CS but decreased the oxidative stress induced by CCl4 in activated hepatic stellated cells (HSC). Among others, this antifibrotic effect was associated with the attenuation of TGF-β/Smad, Wnt/β-catenin, MAPK, and mitochondrial signaling pathways [74]. Recent investigations have shown that Sir2 enzyme members, collectively called sirtuins, are involved in CS associated with liver diseases. Sirtuin 6 (SIRT6), an enzyme that promotes resistance to DNA damage and oxidative stress, plays a central role in the CS induced by ROS and TGF-β signaling in HCC cells [75]. In this report, ROS and TGF-β upregulated SIRT6 expression by inducing sustained activation of extracelular signal-regulated kinase (ERK) and Smad pathways. Upregulated SIRT6 not only abrogated the inducing effect of TGF-β and ROS on CS but was also required for the ERK pathway to suppress p16 and p21 expression. Additionally, upregulation of SIRT6 promoted HCC cell tumorigenicity and contributed to the inhibitory effect of the ERK pathway on cellular senescence. This feedback loop activation integrated by SIRT6 and TGF-β has the potential to modulate both tumorigenicity and senescence and represents a clear example of the molecular complexity around senescence activation. Another investigation group demonstrated that SIRT1, an enzyme that deacetylates nonhistone proteins and allows mammalian cell survival under oxidative stress, is downregulated in aged and middle-aged mice. This condition increased mice susceptibility to the effect produced by chronic alcohol consumption and exacerbated alcoholic liver injury and fibrosis in hepatocytes and hepatic stellate cells [76]. This evidence clearly reveals that the senescence and ROS pair in the liver of elderly patients boosts alcohol liver disease, likely by the modification of liver metabolic functions. This proposal is in accordance with a recent report of Cyp2e1 as a central player in aging-dependent hepatic steatosis, apoptosis, and fibrosis. The investigation demonstrated that Cyp2e1 increased the production of reactive nitrogen species and ROS in aged mice; as a result, high levels of lipid peroxidation, oxidative protein modifications, oxidative DNA damage, and inflammation were found. These changes were absent or decreased in aged Cyp2e1-null mice [77]. In the serum of patients with nonalcoholic steatohepatitis (NASH) and NASH-related HCC, oxidative stress correlated with the levels of NASH activity markers, while the antioxidative function was preserved in younger patients as well as in patients with a well-preserved liver function; in contrast, patients with NASH-related HCC tended to be older and exhibited a diminished antioxidative function [78]. In addition to the complexities involved with senescence and ROS in liver diseases, there is evidence of SIRT1 and Cyp2e1 as possible targets for preventing aging-related liver disease.

Senescence induction has also been another means for researchers to determine the efficiency of chemotherapeutic agents against cancer. Most of these agents are strong oxidative stress inducers such as cisplatin. In a recent study, this compound promoted a senescent phenotype in HCC cell lines dependent on p53 and p21 activation and intracellular ROS generation [79]. Although senescence activation appears to be a natural consequence of oxidative stress induction, ROS generation may dictate different cellular consequences depending on the overall concentration at steady-state levels and site of generation [80]. In support of this, an advanced investigation has conferred an important role for ROS production and its participation as a decisive factor in the progression and aggressiveness of cancer [81], and has also raised the complexity of the senescence and ROS pair. Investigators reported that the normally high potential for melanoma cells to form subcutaneous tumors is limited after intravenous or intrasplenic transplantation; this occurs because metastatic cells experience a charge of oxidative stress in the blood and visceral organs, which is not present in established subcutaneous tumors. To overcome that barrier, cells undergo reversible metabolic changes during metastasis that increase their capability to withstand oxidative stress. It was found that mitochondrial membrane potential, mass, and ROS levels declined more in circulating metastatic cells compared to subcutaneous tumors, raising the possibility that mitochondrial function is reduced in circulating melanoma cells in an effort to reduce ROS generation [81]. During the normal aging process, mitochondrial metabolic changes are implicated in the induction and maintenance of CS [82]. While the investigation did not show whether oxidative stress also limits the initiation and early growth of primary cutaneous cancer cells [81], it is reasonable to hypothesize that senescence activation and/or ROS generation are determinant factors of the appearance and progression of different multifocal HCC types. This intriguing hypothesis stems from a proposal that multifocal HCCs are either from an HCC of multicentric origin or HCC of intrahepatic metastasis [83]. Thus, in this scenario, ROS may modulate CS activation in the HCC microenvironment. As a result, senescence and ROS may be the decisive molecular pair to establish the outcome of multifocal HCC. This hypothetical proposal also raises the question of whether the appearance of senescence/ROS is a transitory, sporadic, or specific event of a determined HCC development stage. We have recently shown that, concomitant to the HCC development induced by diethylnitrosamine, there is also a chronological appearance of CS [69]; however, its association with ROS generation and effect on the outcome of multifocal HCC type has not been investigated. This is an interesting and comprehensive proposal worth investigating.

3. Is cellular senescence important in the development of hepatic diseases?

Aging changes the biological processes in many organs and tissues of mammalians, leading to the development of age-associated diseases and aberrant body homeostasis. Nearly 13% of the population in the United States is over the age of 65 years; this percentage and the number of elderly people will increase substantially over the next 50 years [84]. Although the aging process does not cause death, elderly people appear to be predisposed to a variety of diseases; therefore, aging facilitates the onset and/or progression of various pathologies including diseases of the liver [84]. The ability to withstand hepatic insult decreases each decade, including those associated with high triglyceride levels, nonalcoholic fatty liver diseases, and HCC [85–87]. The percentage of deaths caused by liver diseases increases dramatically in humans over the age of 45 years. Accordingly, age is a critical determinant in the outcome of hepatitis C infection [88] and liver transplantation [89]. However, the most dramatic effect of aging on the liver is its delayed and/or reduced proliferation after a loss of mass from a surgical or chemical injury [90–92]. Based on these correlations, it has been suggested that elderly people are predisposed to liver diseases. The livers of young individuals regenerate after these treatments and maintain homeostasis; conversely, there is a dramatically reduced regeneration of the livers of older people. The clinical outcome of human acute liver injury is also partially dependent on the potential for hepatic regeneration. In older people, there is a higher incidence of acute liver failure and a higher mortality with acute hepatitis A [93, 94]. In a cohort of patients with acute liver failure secondary to viral hepatitis, age was an independent predictor of a poor outcome, with the worst outcomes in people over the age of 50 years [95]. Wong et al. and Poynard et al. were among the first to demonstrate that age at infection was a major risk factor for subsequent fibrosis progression and that the rate of fibrosis progression accelerated with increasing age [96, 97]. Studies of other liver diseases have demonstrated similar findings. Age is an independent risk factor for poor outcomes in primary biliary cirrhosis (PBC) in addition to the presence of portal hypertension and impaired liver function [98]. Similarly, age, independent of bilirubin, prothrombin time, and renal function, predicted the outcome in patients with alcoholic hepatitis [99]. There is some evidence that age may influence disease progression in nonalcoholic fatty liver disease (NAFLD) [100, 101].

The role of CS in diverse chronic liver diseases has come into recent research. The structure of hepatocytes changes with age. The volume of hepatocytes increases with development and maturation but declines with senescence [84]. The relative volumes of hepatocyte organelles also change during aging. The universal change in diagnostic liver biopsy specimens is the age-related cytoplasmic accumulation of highly oxidized insoluble protein lipofuscin or age pigment, which in turn reflects a concomitant increase in the volume of the dense body compartment [102]. Accelerated hepatocyte aging and the accumulation of senescent hepatocytes have been found in diverse chronic liver disorders [103–108]. Furthermore, the studies have shown that the increased proportion of senescent hepatocytes is associated independently with increased fibrosis stage, impaired hepatic function, and an adverse liver-related outcome including liver-related death [103–109]. However, it is still unknown whether hepatocyte senescence contributes causally to fibrosis progression, declining hepatic function, or the increased risk of an adverse liver-related outcome.

3.1. Hepatic fibrosis

Hepatic fibrosis is a common pathological consequence of chronic liver diseases and results from the progressive accumulation of an excess quantity of extracellular matrix (ECM) tissue. In many patients, continuous liver parenchyma insult ultimately leads to cirrhosis [110]. The ECM accumulation during chronic liver injury is caused by a heterogeneous population of myofibroblasts derived mainly from hepatic stellate cells and from resident fibroblasts. Myofibroblasts are highly proliferative cells with enhanced survival that migrate and accumulate at sites of liver damage in response to a liver insult that caused a wide variety of growth factors, cytokines, and lipid mediators. Recently, many studies have observed that the presence of an increased proportion of senescent hepatocytes is associated with an increased fibrosis stage. This results in impaired hepatic function and an adverse liver-related outcome, including liver-related death [103, 104, 106–108].

3.2. Cirrhosis and HCC

In humans, cirrhosis is induced by a variety of liver diseases. Regardless of its etiology, cirrhosis evolves slowly over many years, and chronic hepatocyte death and renewal are major predisposing factors [111]. Cirrhosis is associated with life-threatening complications due to a decreased functional parenchymal reserve and altered hepatic blood flow. A recent report by WHO indicates that cirrhosis accounts for 170,000 deaths in Europe per year [110]. The cellular growth arrest and CS appear to be in a pro-fibrotic state. There is existing research on the relation between cirrhosis and telomere shortening, showing that telomere shortening is a marker of cirrhosis and correlates with senescence-associated β-galactosidase in 84% of cirrhosis samples, specifically in hepatocytes [110]. CS contributes to age-related tissue dysfunction, macroH2A1, and a variant of histone H2A. CS is also a marker of senescence-associated heterochromatic foci that synergizes with DNA methylation to silence tumor-suppressor genes in human fibroblasts. MacroH2A1, a variant of histone H2A, is a marker of senescence-associated heterochromatic foci that synergizes with DNA methylation to silence tumor-suppressor genes in human fibroblasts. In a recent study, Borghesan et al. investigated the relationship between macroH2A1 splice variants, macroH2A1.1 and macroH2A1.2, and liver carcinogenesis. It was found that protein levels of both macroH2A1 isoforms were increased in the livers of very elderly rodents and humans, and were strong immunohistochemical markers of human cirrhosis and HCC [112].

3.3. Chronic hepatitis B

Chronic hepatitis B virus (HBV) infection can lead to the development of chronic hepatitis, cirrhosis, and HCC. HBV infection is associated with age, cell cycle arrest, and CS. In a recent study, the authors assessed the HBV antigen production in relation to cell cycle arrest and CS *in vitro* using hepG2 and hepG2.2.15 cell lines [113].The authors found that cell cycle arrest induced *in vitro* by the addition of H_2O_2 caused increased levels of supernatant HBsAg and HBV DNA and increased expression of HBcAg. In contrast, there was no observed effect on HBsAg or HBV DNA production in senescent cells, with only a minor increase in cytoplasmic HBcAg staining [113].Widespread telomere shortening is consistent with accelerated aging in chronic HBV [114].

3.4. Chronic hepatitis C

Chronic infection with hepatitis C virus (HCV) affects approximately 170 million people around the world. Moreover, 20% of these affected people develop cirrhosis and are at great risk to develop HCC. An increased risk of HCV-related cirrhosis is associated with hepatic steatosis, older age, and higher alcohol consumption [88, 115]. It has been reported that during chronic HCV infection, telomere shortening is present in liver tissue [116], likely due to increased hepatocyte turnover. Critically short telomeres trigger replicative senescence. Marshall et al. found a strong correlation between hepatocyte G1 arrest, dysfunctional hepatic regeneration, and increased cirrhosis in patients with chronic HCV. They showed increased hepatocyte cell cycle arrest measured by the expression of the mini-chromosome maintenance protein 2 (Mcm-2) in liver biopsy samples. The researchers also found that p21 expressed predominantly in hepatocytes and it was correlated with the stage of fibrosis [107].

3.5. Nonalcohol-related fatty liver disease (NAFLD)

NAFLD is a leading cause of chronic liver disease worldwide [117], which presents a wide range of liver disorders including simple steatosis, steatohepatitis, cirrhosis, and HCC [117]. In ob/ob mice, NAFLD is associated with an increased expression of the cell cycle inhibitor p21 and impaired liver regeneration [118]. The combination of impaired regeneration and increased incidence of cancer in NAFLD suggests accelerated aging. In the literature, NAFLD has been separately described by the appearance of premature telomere shortening, increased hepatocyte nuclear area, advanced fibrosis, and p21 expression [103, 104]. Recently, Aravinthan et al. performed a study on 105 archived formalin-fixed paraffin-embedded liver needle biopsy specimens from 70 patients within the spectrum of NAFLD, and 43 liver needle biopsies at the time of liver transplantation from age- and sex-matched donor livers served as controls. In this study, the authors found a close correlation between hepatic steatosis and short telomeres; additionally, the proportion of hepatocytes with DNA damage identified by the presence of γ-H2AX increased in parallel with steatosis grade. The authors suggested that the accumulation of fat in hepatocytes causes DNA damage and telomere erosion, possibly mediated by oxidative stress. A critically short telomere and a break in double-stranded DNA lead to CS and permanent cell cycle arrest. The authors also found a pattern of predominant hepatocyte G1/S phase cell cycle arrest in NAFLD, with an increased expression of Mcm-2 compared to a normal liver. Furthermore, there was increased expression of the p21 protein. A striking feature was the association of p21 expression with the fibrosis stage, which suggests an accumulation of senescent hepatocytes with disease progression [105].

3.6. Alcohol-related liver disease

Alcohol-related liver disease (ALD) is one of the leading causes of liver-related morbidity and mortality in the world. ALD encompasses a broad spectrum of liver injury from simple steatosis to alcohol-related hepatitis, cirrhosis, and HCC. The pathophysiology of ALD is a complex phenomenon; however, oxidative stress is an important factor in the disease since alcohol consumption increases the production of ROS and diminishes cellular antioxidant levels [119]. The validity of clinical criteria in predicting outcomes in ALD has been studied. In one study, it was shown that the increase of the hepatocyte nuclear area was related to hepatic dysfunction and suggests hepatocyte senescence, since nuclear enlargement is a recognized morphological characteristic of CS [120]. In contrast, irreversible cell arrest that limits the proliferative potential of cell is a hallmark of CS and is mediated by p21 [121]. Thus, p21 has a vital role in the stability of cell cycle arrest and the induction of senescence [121].

3.7. Senolytic drugs

The accumulation of senescent cells in tissues and organs contributes to age-related diseases; however, the presence of radiations or genotoxic agents may contribute to the development of senescence phenotype. This accumulation is important because senescent cells contribute to alterations in the microenvironment. This can support conditions for diseases such as cancer to develop, but senescent cell quantity is important for organ function in the case of aging.

Senolytic agents may be used for clearance of senescent cells in the organs. Chang et al. used ABT263, a specific inhibitor of apoptosis genes BCL2 and BCL2L1, to selectively induce apoptosis in senescent cells in culture. They carried out experiments using a mouse model with known p16-3 MR and administered ABT263 to mice and observed that p16-positive senescent cells were depleted in bone marrow, lung, and muscle tissue via apoptosis. The data demonstrate that ABT263 is a senolytic drug that acts in a highly specific manner on various tissues to target senescent cells both in culture and *in vivo*. These findings significantly advance clinical targeting of cell senescence [122].

4. Conclusion

Until now, the role of CS is poorly understood and little studied in hepatology. There are major implications for hepatology in the field of fibrosis and cancer, and liver chronic diseases. Further investigation into the molecular basis of senescence in liver diseases is necessary, and the collaboration between basic and clinical researchers is fundamental to arrive to better diagnosis and treatment.

Acknowledgements

This book chapter was supported by grant No 83710 from CONACyT.

Author details

Ruth Pacheco Rivera[1], Jaime Arellanes Robledo[2] and Jesús Serrano Luna[3*]

*Address all correspondence to: jjserrano07@yahoo.com.mx

1 Departamento de Bioquímica, Escuela Nacional de Ciencias Biológicas del Instituto Politécnico Nacional, Ciudad de México, México

2 Catedras CONACyT, Instituto Nacional de Medicina Genómica, Ciudad de México, México

3 Departamento de Biología Celular, Centro de Investigación y de Estudios Avanzados del IPN, Ciudad de México, México

References

[1] Lopez-Otin C, et al. The hallmarks of aging. Cell. 2013;**153**(6):1194-1217

[2] Campisi J, d'Adda di Fagagna F. Cellular senescence: When bad things happen to good cells. Nature Reviews Molecular Cell Biology. 2007;**8**(9):729-740

[3] Sahin E, DePinho RA. Axis of ageing: Telomeres, p53 and mitochondria. Nature Reviews Molecular Cell Biology. 2012;**13**(6):397-404

[4] Sedelnikova OA, et al. Senescing human cells and ageing mice accumulate DNA lesions with unrepairable double-strand breaks. Nature Cell Biology. 2004;**6**(2):168-170

[5] Chen QM, et al. Uncoupling the senescent phenotype from telomere shortening in hydrogen peroxide-treated fibroblasts. Experimental Cell Research. 2001;**265**(2):294-303

[6] Parrinello S, et al. Oxygen sensitivity severely limits the replicative lifespan of murine fibroblasts. Nature Cell Biology. 2003;**5**(8):741-747

[7] Cheung AL, Deng W. Telomere dysfunction, genome instability and cancer. Frontiers in Bioscience. 2008;**13**:2075-2090

[8] Sarkisian CJ, et al. Dose-dependent oncogene-induced senescence *in vivo* and its evasion during mammary tumorigenesis. Nature Cell Biology. 2007;**9**(5):493-505

[9] Blagosklonny MV. Cell senescence and hypermitogenic arrest. European Molecular Biology Organization Reports. 2003;**4**(4):358-362

[10] Serrano M, et al. Oncogenic ras provokes premature cell senescence associated with accumulation of p53 and p16INK4a. Cell. 1997;**88**(5):593-602

[11] Degirmenci U, Lei S. Role of lncRNAs in cellular aging. Frontiers in Endocrinology (Lausanne). 2016;**7**:151

[12] Hayflick L, Moorhead PS. The serial cultivation of human diploid cell strains. Experimental Cell Research. 1961;**25**:585-621

[13] Coppe JP, et al. The senescence-associated secretory phenotype: The dark side of tumor suppression. Annual Review of Pathology. 2010;**5**:99-118

[14] Dimri GP, et al. A biomarker that identifies senescent human cells in culture and in aging skin *in vivo*. Proceedings of the National Academy of Sciences of the United States of America. 1995;**92**(20):9363-9367

[15] Campisi J. Cellular senescence as a tumor-suppressor mechanism. Trends in Cell Biology. 2001;**11**(11):S27-31

[16] Shimi T, et al. The role of nuclear lamin B1 in cell proliferation and senescence. Genes & Development. 2011;**25**(24):2579-2593

[17] Freund A, et al. Inflammatory networks during cellular senescence: Causes and consequences. Trends in Molecular Medicine. 2010;**16**(5):238-246

[18] Munoz-Espin D, Serrano M. Cellular senescence: From physiology to pathology. Nature Reviews Molecular Cell Biology. 2014;**15**(7):482-496

[19] Kim WY, Sharpless NE. The regulation of INK4/ARF in cancer and aging. Cell. 2006;**127**(2):265-275

[20] Webley KM, Shorthouse AJ, Royds JA. Effect of mutation and conformation on the function of p53 in colorectal cancer. The Journal of Pathology. 2000;**191**(4):361-367

[21] d'Adda di Fagagna F, et al. A DNA damage checkpoint response in telomere-initiated senescence. Nature. 2003;**426**(6963):194-198

[22] Dyson N. The regulation of E2F by pRB-family proteins. Genes & Development. 1998;**12**(15):2245-2262

[23] Haupt Y, et al. Mdm2 promotes the rapid degradation of p53. Nature. 1997;**387**(6630): 296-299

[24] Wang L, et al. Requirement of mitogen-activated protein kinase kinase 3 (MKK3) for activation of p38alpha and p38delta MAPK isoforms by TGF-beta 1 in murine mesangial cells. Journal of Biological Chemistry. 2002;**277**(49):47257-47262

[25] Iwasa H, Han J, Ishikawa F. Mitogen-activated protein kinase p38 defines the common senescence-signalling pathway. Genes Cells. 2003;**8**(2):131-144

[26] Ishikawa Y, et al. Regulation of Bax translocation through phosphorylation at Ser-70 of Bcl-2 by MAP kinase in NO-induced neuronal apoptosis. Molecular and Cellular Neuroscience. 2003;**24**(2):451-459

[27] Hu X, et al. A functional genomic approach identifies FAL1 as an oncogenic long noncoding RNA that associates with BMI1 and represses p21 expression in cancer. Cancer Cell. 2014;**26**(3):344-357

[28] Zhong X, Hu X, Zhang L. Oncogenic long noncoding RNA FAL1 in human cancer. Molecular and Cellular Oncology. 2015;**2**(2):e977154

[29] Shi Y, et al. Downregulated long noncoding RNA BANCR promotes the proliferation of colorectal cancer cells via downregualtion of p21 expression. PLoS One. 2015;**10**(4):e0122679

[30] Dimitrova N, et al. LincRNA-p21 activates p21 in cis to promote polycomb target gene expression and to enforce the G1/S checkpoint. Molecular Cell. 2014;**54**(5):777-790

[31] Tripathi V, et al. The nuclear-retained noncoding RNA MALAT1 regulates alternative splicing by modulating SR splicing factor phosphorylation. Molecular Cell. 2010;**39**(6):925-938

[32] Abdelmohsen K, et al. 7SL RNA represses p53 translation by competing with HuR. Nucleic Acids Research. 2014;**42**(15):10099-10111

[33] Lazorthes S, et al. A vlincRNA participates in senescence maintenance by relieving H2AZ-mediated repression at the INK4 locus. Nature Communications. 2015;**6**:5971

[34] Kotake Y, et al. Long non-coding RNA ANRIL is required for the PRC2 recruitment to and silencing of p15(INK4B) tumor suppressor gene. Oncogene. 2011;**30**(16):1956-1962

[35] Yap KL, et al. Molecular interplay of the noncoding RNA ANRIL and methylated histone H3 lysine 27 by polycomb CBX7 in transcriptional silencing of INK4a. Molecular Cell. 2010;**38**(5):662-674

[36] Montes M, et al. The lncRNA MIR31HG regulates p16(INK4A) expression to modulate senescence. Nature Communications. 2015;**6**:6967

[37] Kumar PP, et al. Coordinated control of senescence by lncRNA and a novel T-box3 co-repressor complex. Elife. 2014;**3**:1-28

[38] Xue M, Chen W, Li X. Urothelial cancer associated 1: A long noncoding RNA with a crucial role in cancer. Journal of Cancer Research and Clinical Oncology. 2016;**142**(7):1407-1419

[39] Wu CL, et al. Senescence-associated long non-coding RNA (SALNR) delays oncogene-induced senescence through NF90 regulation. Journal of Biological Chemistry. 2015;**290**(50):30175-30192

[40] Arnoult N, Van Beneden A, Decottignies A. Telomere length regulates TERRA levels through increased trimethylation of telomeric H3K9 and HP1alpha. Nature Structural & Molecular Biology. 2012;**19**(9):948-956

[41] Taft RJ, et al. Non-coding RNAs: Regulators of disease. The Journal of Pathology. 2010;**220**(2):126-139

[42] Beausejour CM, et al. Reversal of human cellular senescence: Roles of the p53 and p16 pathways. European Molecular Biology Organization Journal. 2003;**22**(16):4212-4222

[43] Narita M, et al. A novel role for high-mobility group a proteins in cellular senescence and heterochromatin formation. Cell. 2006;**126**(3):503-514

[44] Ye ZW, et al. Oxidative stress, redox regulation and diseases of cellular differentiation. Biochimica et Biophysica Acta. 2015;**1850**(8):1607-1621

[45] Sid B, Verrax J, Calderon PB. Role of oxidative stress in the pathogenesis of alcohol-induced liver disease. Free Radical Research. 2013;**47**(11):894-904

[46] Yang HY, Lee TH. Antioxidant enzymes as redox-based biomarkers: A brief review. BMB Reports. 2015;**48**(4):200-208

[47] Bouayed J, Bohn T. Exogenous antioxidants-double-edged swords in cellular redox state: Health beneficial effects at physiologic doses versus deleterious effects at high doses. Oxidative Medicine and Cellular Longevity. 2010;**3**(4):228-237

[48] Alfadda AA, Sallam RM. Reactive oxygen species in health and disease. Journal of Biomedicine and Biotechnology. 2012;**2012**:936486

[49] Ha HL, et al. Oxidative stress and antioxidants in hepatic pathogenesis. World Journal of Gastroenterology. 2010;**16**(48):6035-6043

[50] Mari M, et al. Redox control of liver function in health and disease. Antioxidants & Redox Signaling. 2010;**12**(11):1295-1331

[51] Serviddio G, Bellanti F, Vendemiale G. Free radical biology for medicine: Learning from nonalcoholic fatty liver disease. Free Radical Biology and Medicine. 2013;**65**:952-968

[52] Parola M, Robino G. Oxidative stress-related molecules and liver fibrosis. Journal of Hepatology. 2001;**35**(2):297-306

[53] Nair J, et al. High urinary excretion of lipid peroxidation-derived DNA damage in patients with cancer-prone liver diseases. Mutation Research. 2010;**683**(1-2):23-28

[54] Lu T, Finkel T. Free radicals and senescence. Experimental Cell Research. 2008;**314**(9):1918-1922

[55] Chen Q, et al. Oxidative DNA damage and senescence of human diploid fibroblast cells. Proceedings of the National Academy of Sciences of the United States of America. 1995;**92**(10):4337-4341

[56] von Zglinicki T, Oxidative stress shortens telomeres. Trends in Biochemical Sciences. 2002;**27**(7):339-344

[57] Rodier F, Campisi J. Four faces of cellular senescence. Journal of Cell Biology. 2011;**192**(4):547-556

[58] Krizhanovsky V, et al. Senescence of activated stellate cells limits liver fibrosis. Cell. 2008;**134**(4):657-667

[59] Passos JF, et al. Feedback between p21 and reactive oxygen production is necessary for cell senescence. Molecular Systems Biology. 2010;**6**:347

[60] Takahashi A, et al. Mitogenic signalling and the p16INK4a-Rb pathway cooperate to enforce irreversible cellular senescence. Nature Cell Biology. 2006;**8**(11):1291-1297

[61] Lee AC, et al. Ras proteins induce senescence by altering the intracellular levels of reactive oxygen species. Journal of Biological Chemistry. 1999;**274**(12):7936-7940

[62] Macip S, et al. Influence of induced reactive oxygen species in p53-mediated cell fate decisions. Molecular and Cellular Biology. 2003;**23**(23):8576-8585

[63] Rolo AP, Teodoro JS, Palmeira CM. Role of oxidative stress in the pathogenesis of nonalcoholic steatohepatitis. Free Radical Biology and Medicine. 2012;**52**(1):59-69

[64] Paradis V, et al. Replicative senescence in normal liver, chronic hepatitis C, and hepatocellular carcinomas. Human Pathology. 2001;**32**(3):327-332

[65] Ramakrishna G, et al. From cirrhosis to hepatocellular carcinoma: New molecular insights on inflammation and cellular senescence. Liver Cancer. 2013;**2**(3-4):367-383

[66] Schnabl B, et al. Replicative senescence of activated human hepatic stellate cells is accompanied by a pronounced inflammatory but less fibrogenic phenotype. Hepatology. 2003;**37**(3):653-664

[67] Kang TW, et al. Senescence surveillance of pre-malignant hepatocytes limits liver cancer development. Nature. 2011;**479**(7374):547-551

[68] Schiffer E, et al. Gefitinib, an EGFR inhibitor, prevents hepatocellular carcinoma development in the rat liver with cirrhosis. Hepatology. 2005;**41**(2):307-314

[69] Pacheco-Rivera R, et al. Double staining of beta-galactosidase with fibrosis and cancer markers reveals the chronological appearance of senescence in liver carcinogenesis induced by diethylnitrosamine. Toxicology Letters. 2016;**241**:19-31

[70] Verna L, Whysner J, Williams GM. N-nitrosodiethylamine mechanistic data and risk assessment: Bioactivation, DNA-adduct formation, mutagenicity, and tumor initiation. Pharmacology & Therapeutics. 1996;**71**(1-2):57-81

[71] Aravinthan A, et al. Selective insulin resistance in hepatocyte senescence. Experimental Cell Research. 2015;**331**(1):38-45

[72] Aravinthan A, et al. The senescent hepatocyte gene signature in chronic liver disease. Experimental Gerontology. 2014;**60**:37-45

[73] Borkham-Kamphorst E, et al. The anti-fibrotic effects of CCN1/CYR61 in primary portal myofibroblasts are mediated through induction of reactive oxygen species resulting in cellular senescence, apoptosis and attenuated TGF-beta signaling. Biochimica et Biophysica Acta. 2014;**1843**(5):902-914

[74] Zhang X, et al. Potent effects of dioscin against liver fibrosis. Scientific Reports. 2015;**5**: 9713

[75] Feng XX, et al. Sirtuin 6 promotes transforming growth factor-beta1/H2O2/HOCl-mediated enhancement of hepatocellular carcinoma cell tumorigenicity by suppressing cellular senescence. Cancer Science. 2015;**106**(5):559-566

[76] Ramirez T, et al. Aging aggravates alcoholic liver injury and fibrosis in mice by downregulating sirtuin 1 expression. Journal of Hepatology. 2017;**66**(3):601-609

[77] Abdelmegeed MA, et al. Cytochrome P450-2E1 promotes aging-related hepatic steatosis, apoptosis and fibrosis through increased nitroxidative stress. Free Radical Biology and Medicine. 2016;**91**:188-202

[78] Shimomura Y, et al. The serum oxidative/anti-oxidative stress balance becomes dysregulated in patients with non-alcoholic steatohepatitis associated with hepatocellular carcinoma. Internal Medicine. 2017;**56**(3):243-251

[79] Qu K, et al. Reactive oxygen species generation is essential for cisplatin-induced accelerated senescence in hepatocellular carcinoma. Frontiers in Medicine. 2014;**8**(2):227-235

[80] Panieri E, et al. Reactive oxygen species generated in different compartments induce cell death, survival, or senescence. Free Radical Biology and Medicine. 2013;**57**:176-187

[81] Piskounova E, et al. Oxidative stress inhibits distant metastasis by human melanoma cells. Nature. 2015;**527**(7577):186-191

[82] Correia-Melo C, Passos JF. Mitochondria: Are they causal players in cellular senescence? Biochimica et Biophysica Acta. 2015;**1847**(11):1373-1379

[83] Feo F, Pascale RM. Multifocal hepatocellular carcinoma: Intrahepatic metastasis or multicentric carcinogenesis? Annals of Translational Medicine. 2015;**3**(1):4

[84] Schmucker DL. Age-related changes in liver structure and function: Implications for disease ? Experimental Gerontology. 2005;**40**(8-9):650-659

[85] Cuadrado A, et al. Non-alcoholic steatohepatitis (NASH) and hepatocellular carcinoma. Obesity Surgery. 2005;**15**(3):442-446

[86] Cankurtaran M, et al. Serum vitamin-E levels and its relation to clinical features in nonalcoholic fatty liver disease with elevated ALT levels. Acta Gastroenterolgica Belgica. 2006;**69**(1):5-11

[87] Blouin K, et al. Contribution of age and declining androgen levels to features of the metabolic syndrome in men. Metabolism. 2005;**54**(8):1034-1040

[88] Poynard T, et al. Rates and risk factors of liver fibrosis progression in patients with chronic hepatitis c. Journal of Hepatology. 2001;**34**(5):730-739

[89] Keswani SC, Rosenberg B, Hoke A. The use of GAP-43 mRNA quantification in high throughput screening of putative neuroprotective agents in dorsal root ganglion cultures. Journal of Neuroscience Methods. 2004;**136**(2):193-195

[90] Fry M, et al. Delayed and reduced cell replication and diminishing levels of DNA polymerase-alpha in regenerating liver of aging mice. Journal of Cellular Physiology. 1984;**118**(3):225-232

[91] Timchenko NA, et al. Regenerating livers of old rats contain high levels of C/EBPalpha that correlate with altered expression of cell cycle associated proteins. Nucleic Acids Research. 1998;**26**(13):3293-3299

[92] Iakova P, Awad SS, Timchenko NA. Aging reduces proliferative capacities of liver by switching pathways of C/EBPalpha growth arrest. Cell. 2003;**113**(4):495-506

[93] Forbes A, Williams R. Increasing age--an important adverse prognostic factor in hepatitis A virus infection. Journal of the Royal College of Physicians of London. 1988;**22**(4):237-239

[94] Forbes A, Williams R. Changing epidemiology and clinical aspects of hepatitis A. British Medical Bulletin. 1990;**46**(2):303-318

[95] Dhiman RK, et al. Early indicators of prognosis in fulminant hepatic failure: An assessment of the Model for End-Stage Liver Disease (MELD) and King's College Hospital criteria. Liver Transplantation. 2007;**13**(6):814-821

[96] Wong V, et al. Importance of age in chronic hepatitis C virus infection. Journal of Viral Hepatitis. 1997;**4**(4):255-264

[97] Poynard T. Interferon alpha in hepatitis C: A cytokine for reducing fibrosis progression. European Cytokine Network. 1997;**8**(3):319-320

[98] Goudie BM, et al. Risk factors and prognosis in primary biliary cirrhosis. The American Journal of Gastroenterology. 1989;**84**(7):713-716

[99] Forrest EH, et al. Analysis of factors predictive of mortality in alcoholic hepatitis and derivation and validation of the Glasgow alcoholic hepatitis score. Gut. 2005;**54**(8):1174-1179

[100] Ratziu V, et al. Liver fibrosis in overweight patients. Gastroenterology. 2000;**118**(6): 1117-1123

[101] Angulo P, et al. Independent predictors of liver fibrosis in patients with nonalcoholic steatohepatitis. Hepatology. 1999;**30**(6):1356-1362

[102] Schmucker DL, Sachs H. Quantifying dense bodies and lipofuscin during aging: A morphologist's perspective. Archives of Gerontology and Geriatrics. 2002;**34**(3):249-261

[103] Nakajima T, et al. Premature telomere shortening and impaired regenerative response in hepatocytes of individuals with NAFLD. Liver international. 2006;**26**(1):23-31

[104] Richardson MM, et al. Progressive fibrosis in nonalcoholic steatohepatitis: Association with altered regeneration and a ductular reaction. Gastroenterology. 2007;**133**(1):80-90

[105] Aravinthan A, et al. Hepatocyte expression of the senescence marker p21 is linked to fibrosis and an adverse liver-related outcome in alcohol-related liver disease. PLoS One. 2013;**8**(9):e72904

[106] Aravinthan A, et al. Hepatocyte senescence predicts progression in non-alcohol-related fatty liver disease. Journal of Hepatology. 2013;**58**(3):549-556

[107] Marshall A, et al. Relation between hepatocyte G1 arrest, impaired hepatic regeneration, and fibrosis in chronic hepatitis C virus infection. Gastroenterology. 2005;**128**(1):33-42

[108] Wood MJ, et al. Ductular reaction in hereditary hemochromatosis: The link between hepatocyte senescence and fibrosis progression. Hepatology. 2014;**59**(3):848-857

[109] Gonzalez-Reimers E, et al. Hepatocyte and nuclear areas and fatty infiltration of the liver in chronic alcoholic liver disease. Drug and Alcohol Dependence. 1988;**22**(3):195-203

[110] Mallat A, Lotersztajn S. Cellular mechanisms of tissue fibrosis. 5. Novel insights into liver fibrosis. American Journal of Physiology Cell Physiology. 2013;**305**(8):C789-799

[111] Friedman SL. Liver fibrosis - from bench to bedside. Journal of Hepatology. 2003;**38 Suppl 1**:S38-S53

[112] Borghesan M, et al. DNA hypomethylation and histone variant macroH2A1 synergistically attenuate chemotherapy-induced senescence to promote hepatocellular carcinoma progression. Cancer Research. 2016;**76**(3):594-606

[113] Tachtatzis PM, et al. Correction: Chronic hepatitis B virus infection: The relation between hepatitis B antigen expression, telomere length, senescence, inflammation and fibrosis. PLoS One. 2015;**10**(7):e0134315

[114] Kim H, et al. Large liver cell change in hepatitis B virus-related liver cirrhosis. Hepatology. 2009;**50**(3):752-762

[115] Adinolfi LE, et al. Steatosis accelerates the progression of liver damage of chronic hepatitis C patients and correlates with specific HCV genotype and visceral obesity. Hepatology. 2001;**33**(6):1358-1364

[116] Miura N, et al. Progressive telomere shortening and telomerase reactivation during hepatocellular carcinogenesis. Cancer Genetics and Cytogenetics. 1997;**93**(1):56-62

[117] de Alwis NM, Day CP. Non-alcoholic fatty liver disease: The mist gradually clears. Journal of Hepatology. 2008;**48 Suppl 1**:S104-112

[118] Torbenson M, et al. STAT-3 overexpression and p21 up-regulation accompany impaired regeneration of fatty livers. The American Journal of Pathology. 2002;**161**(1):155-161

[119] O'Shea RS, Dasarathy S, McCullough AJ. Alcoholic liver disease. The American Journal of Gastroenterology. 2010;**105**(1):14-32. quiz 33.

[120] Ben-Porath I, Weinberg RA. The signals and pathways activating cellular senescence. The International Journal of Biochemistry & Cell Biology. 2005;**37**(5):961-976

[121] d'Adda di Fagagna F. Living on a break: Cellular senescence as a DNA-damage response. Nature Reviews Cancer. 2008;**8**(7):512-522

[122] Chang J, et al. Clearance of senescent cells by ABT263 rejuvenates aged hematopoietic stem cells in mice. Nature Medicine. 2016;**22**(1):78-83

Chapter 8

Potential Reduction in Mortality Associated with the Shifts of Population Educational Structures in the Czech Republic

Jitka Rychtaříková and Klára Hulíková Tesárková

Additional information is available at the end of the chapter

http://dx.doi.org/10.5772/intechopen.69635

Abstract

Educational inequalities in mortality are large in Central and Eastern Europe. Mortality levels are particularly high among low educated men as well as women in the Czech Republic. However, differences in male mortality by educational attainment exceed those of females. Two mortality patterns are apparent when dividing the Czech classification of education into four categories—basic, vocational, secondary, and university. Males with basic education experience much higher mortality when compared to their higher educated counterparts. An anomaly in the mortality gradient is observed among women when comparing basic and vocational education. Women with basic education show a rather lower mortality level compared to their vocational counterparts. Three scenarios show how the shifts toward a higher education could contribute to the change in mortality level using temporary life expectancies between ages 30 and 80 for males and females: (a) population structure by sex, age, and education remains the same as from the census 2011; (b) 60% of males having the basic education move into the next higher category (vocational) and 60% of women with basic and vocational education move into the secondary education; and (3) sex age education-specific mortality rates will be shifted upwards by one level.

Keywords: mortality, education attainment, sex-differences, Czech Republic population, scenario

1. Introduction

Kitagawa and Hauser [1] did the first one of the most complete studies of mortality differentials by socioeconomic status (SES) in the United States. They found that higher SES groups exhibited lower rates of all-cause mortality than did lower SES groups. Later on, the Black Report on Inequalities in Health [2] published by the Department of Health and Social Security in the United Kingdom launched debates about widening socioeconomic inequalities in mortality. Significant differentials in mortality by SES had been identified despite a tremendous increase in life expectancy at birth after the World War II. Since then, many studies have pointed out the differences in mortality by socioeconomic status [1, 3–8]. Moreover, time trends in socioeconomic inequalities in mortality have shown a widening of the gap, in relative terms, in Europe as well as in North America [9–12]. Education, occupational status, and income are the most widely used indicators of socioeconomic status. In reality, socioeconomic stratification reflects benefits or returns of a given educational attainment. Therefore, education has become one of the most commonly used indicators of socioeconomic position. The reasons for its use are that educational level can be determined for all individuals (including older people and women). Educational attainment is normally completed by the early adult years and does not change later in life [13]. The educational level can be considered as a proxy not only for the socioeconomic position/class but also because better-educated people lead a healthy lifestyle and can be more efficient consumers of health care. They are also more likely to take advantage of new technologies especially in treatment and prevention [6, 14, 15]. Therefore, the inverse association between education and mortality risk (the gradient) has been evidenced in many studies as well [6, 16–19]. Educational attainment is also a concrete indicator (compared to occupation) for policymakers when deciding the health or social policies and investments [15].

Educational inequalities in mortality are large in Central and Eastern Europe [20]. Mortality levels are particularly high among low educated men as well as women in the Czech Republic. Therefore, we assume that on average, higher levels of schooling cause people to live longer. The main purpose of our study is to find out to what extent the shifts in population structure toward higher education or mortality reduction based on the shifts of death rates toward one higher educational degree will impact on temporary life expectancy between ages 30 and 80. Changes in education-associated excess mortality aimed at lowering the risks present a challenge for social and health policies. For instance, Woolf et al. [21] showed that more lives would be saved by eliminating education-associated excess mortality than by medical advances only.

The contribution will address the following issues: First, to show long-term trends in life expectancy at birth in the Czech Republic,[1] France, and USA. Second, to illustrate differentials in life expectancy at age 30 by education for selected European countries. Third, to present three scenarios that will show how shifts (in population structure or in mortality rates) toward a higher education contribute to the change in all-cause mortality level between ages 30 and 80 using temporary life expectancy indicator.

[1]All results are related to the territory of the current Czech Republic

2. Long-term trends in mortality: The Czech Republic, France, and United States

In 2012, US life expectancy at birth reached 81.2 years for women and 76.4 years for men [22]. These figures can also be found in the Czech Republic in 2015 [23] where women's life expectancy at birth was almost the same reaching 81.4 years and slightly shorter for men with 75.8 years (Czech Republic 2012: men 75.0; women 80.9). However, in the United States, the life expectancy at birth for both women and men is not as long as in France [24]. In 2012, French women lived 4 years longer than their American counterparts—84.8 years versus 81.2 years—and for men, the figures were 78.5 and 76.4 years, respectively. Looking back to the history, more particularly before the World War II, the situation was the reverse and US males and females enjoyed better survival [25]. Since the 1980s, life expectancy has increased much more slowly in the United States compared with France and the lag behind France is widening (**Figure 1a** and **b**).

The American slowdown is especially marked among women. Current US lower life expectancy at birth compared to French one is for instance explained by the fact that although the United States are world leaders in technological and medical innovation, not all inhabitants benefit equally. Unlike Europe, a large proportion of the US population have no health

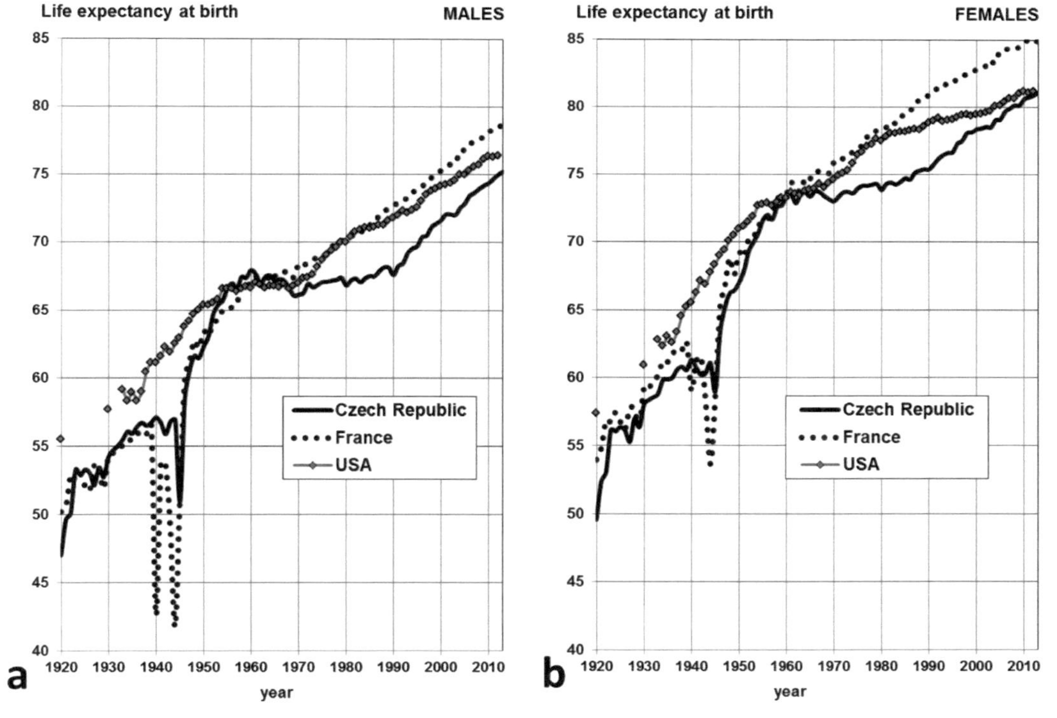

Figure 1. a) Trends in life expectancy at birth since 1920, males. b) Trends in life expectancy at birth since 1920, females.

insurance, and their access to health care is limited [25]. Despite the recent slowdown, US healthcare expenditures exceed those of other high-income countries in Europe [26]. The high cost of US healthcare may to some extent explain the higher levels of mortality compared to the high income population of Europe. In July 2014, The Lancet journal published a series of contributions on the health of Americans [27]. According to the authors, a fragmented healthcare delivery system, social environments (differences in health outcomes according to race, education, region), and individual risk factors (health-related behavior: obesity, smoking, physical inactivity, alcohol use, diets low in fruits, and vegetables) play an important role for length of life.

The Czech Republic manifests four dissimilar stages of mortality development (**Figure 1a** and **b**): before World War II; between World War II and mid-1960s; from the mid-1960s to the mid-1980s; and from the mid-1980s until now [28]. During the interwar period up to the mid-1960s, male and female survival in the Czech Republic was close to the levels observed in France [29]. However, age-specific mortality rates at that time were different in both countries. Before WWII, a high infant mortality rate in the Czech population was counterbalanced by a lower mortality at adult ages. Between World War II and the mid-1960s, the situation reversed and the upward trend of life expectancy at birth accelerated mainly because of the decrease in infant mortality rate, while adult and old age mortality had not changed too much. In the Czech Republic from 1950, all health services were nationalized, provided free of charge, and were accessible to anybody according to the new law. Particular attention was paid to child and mother. The comprehensive network of services was established for children and preventive vaccination and medical check-ups became compulsory. The "health-extensive approach"—a large number of medical staff with limited expenditures for equipment, drugs, and maintenance—was successful in reducing and controlling communicable and infectious diseases. Later on, the emergence of new degenerative diseases required a "health intensive approach" involving specialized training, sophisticated equipment, and expensive procedures and drugs. Despite growing awareness among the medical profession, health systems were not able to adjust to the changing health needs of the population. Therefore, the trend of increased mortality started in the mid-1960s and affected most of the population of Central and Eastern Europe including the Czech Republic. The deterioration was particularly marked for the elderly and middle-aged adults and primarily for men. A substantial part of the mortality increase was attributable to an "epidemic" of heart diseases. To a lesser degree, an increase in cerebrovascular diseases, lung cancer, and cirrhosis of the liver was noticed [29]. For instance, by the mid-1980s, the mortality rate from cardiovascular and cerebrovascular diseases was twice as high in the Czech Republic than in France [29]. It appears that the negative mortality development in the Czech Republic since the mid-1960s can be interpreted as an accumulation of previous problems (relatively high mortality of the elderly) and of inapt solutions for new ones (rising intensity of degenerative diseases). From that time, the gap in life expectancy between the Czech Republic and France or USA began to widen rapidly. Since the mid-1980s a new favorable trend in mortality has appeared in the Czech Republic, a new mortality decline has been initiated [28]. From the medical perspective, the use of cardiovascular drugs and the number of operations such as invasive heart surgery increased considerably. In addition, the structure of treatment shifted from traditional medicines to the new generations of drugs. The surgical and invasive procedures such as coronary artery bypass grafts, valve replacements, and angioplasties have also significantly increased [30]. The period of transition, beginning after 1989 and accompanied by political, economic, social, and behavioral transformations, has had a different impact on health conditions in former socialist countries. The Czech Republic escaped "Eastern European mortality crisis" [31] and its health situation improved more rapidly. However, the time delay of the Czech Republic in the reduction of mortality rate compared to France is too big, and therefore, the recent improvement in survival rates has not diminished the gap between both countries and life expectancies at birth have followed an almost parallel trend.

3. Educational inequality in mortality

Educational attainment plays a central role throughout a life course. In early life, harsh conditions (due to parental socioeconomic status) might impact a later-life mortality risk. However, infant and child mortality fell faster during the twentieth century and also childhood health dramatically improved. Thus, the association between early-life conditions and adult mortality has diminished across cohorts at the aggregate level [12]. Consequently, personal behaviors (diet, smoking, alcoholism, exercise) and the knowledge and the use of health technologies affect adult mortality risk more than early life factors [12].

Everywhere, highly educated adults have lower mortality rates than less educated people. Educational differences in mortality are frequently wider among younger adults compared with their older counterparts. The convergence of differentials by education at later age seems to be more complex, and the explanations vary. The study of Beckett [32] confirms the convergence gradient with age and shows that the protective effect of higher education declines with age because higher educated groups only postpone morbidity toward older age. On the other hand, Masters et al. [12] demonstrate the use of age-period-cohort modeling that educational gap in mortality grows across birth cohorts but not across time periods. Disparities in mortality by education are wider among men than among women. However, recent studies have shown that since the mid-1980s the growing gradient for US all-cause female mortality reflected increasing mortality among low educated women and faster-declining mortality among college-educated women [9].

Increases in all-cause life expectancy at adult ages mask a lot of disparities, including diverging trends, among population groups. Well-educated people live longer and thus represent the potential for reducing future mortality developments. Information on stratification by education of population as well as on mortality differentials can help in promoting and targeting health and social policies.

Figure 2a and **b** presents life expectancy at age 30 by gender in European countries where data on education are available. Educational attainment is classified into three categories (ISCED - The International Standard Classification of Education defined by Eurostat): basic = pre-primary, primary, and lower secondary education (ISCED levels 0–2); secondary = upper secondary and post-secondary non-tertiary education (ISCED levels 3 and 4); and tertiary = first and

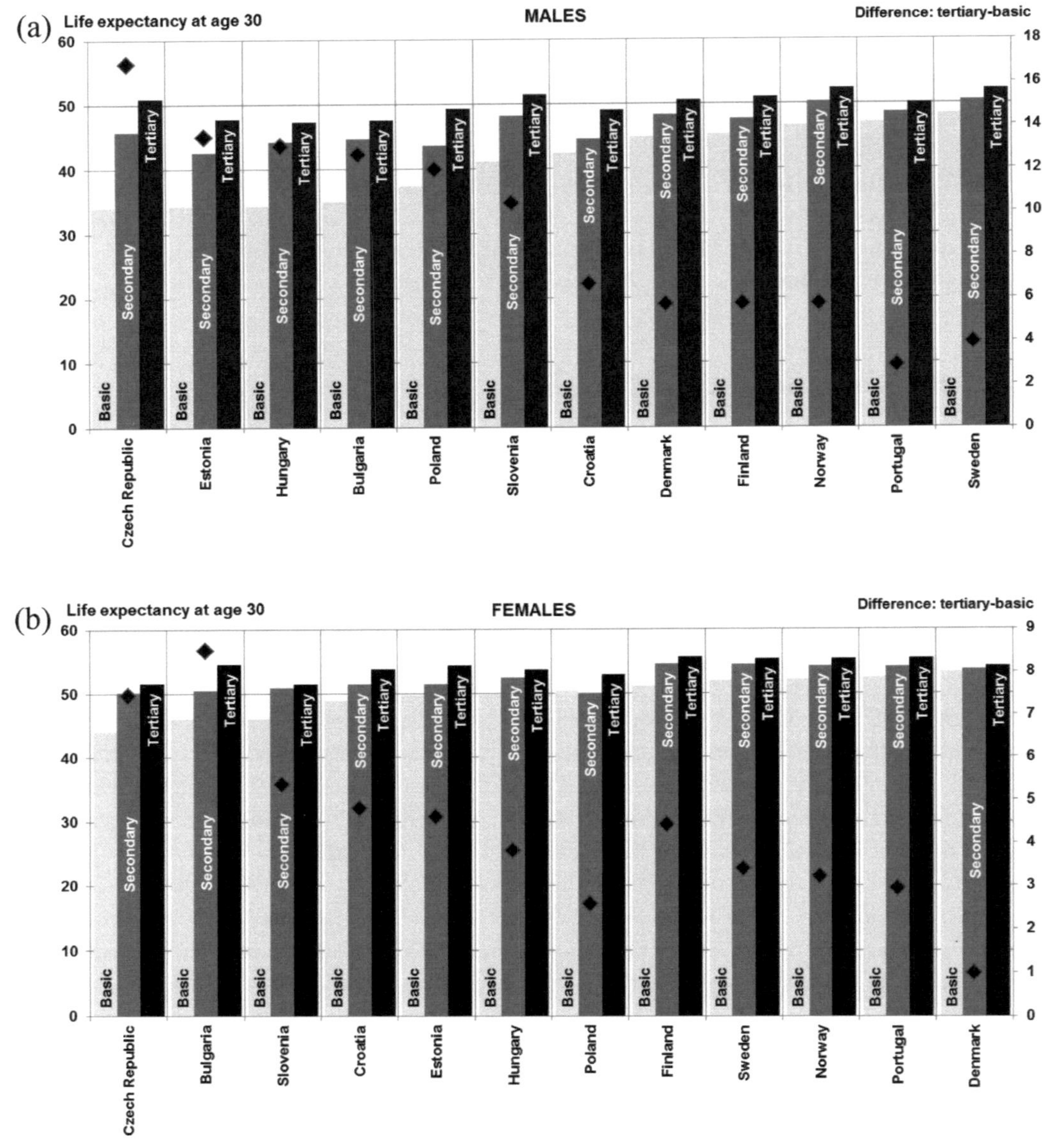

Figure 2. a) Life expectancy at age of 30 according to education level in 2010, males. b) Life expectancy at age of 30 according to education level in 2010, females.

second stage of tertiary education (ISCED levels 5 and 6). In all countries, under the study, highly educated adults experience longer survival (the mean number of remaining years of life beyond age 30 or mean survival duration at age 30 under the mortality conditions of the year in question) than less educated people. The results show variation in survival by educational attainment everywhere. However, former socialist countries show not only shorter life expectancies but also a wide variation in survival by educational attainment for both men and women. The Czech Republic displays a short life expectancy at age 30 for males and females with the lowest education even when compared with countries of higher mortality (Estonia, Hungary, Bulgaria). The difference between life expectancy at 30 of people with the highest and the lowest educational attainment reaches 16.9 years among Czech men compared to 2.9 years in Portugal or 3.9 in Sweden. The gap in Czech female mortality between the highest and the lowest education level is the second high (7.5), after the Bulgarian one (8.5). This phenomenon happens in spite of low social differentiation and universal access to health services. The explanation can be related to the fact that university graduates experienced better health situation because of better working conditions than people with only basic education working in factories with low-tech equipment and therefore in the more detrimental environment. In addition, the lack of knowledge and awareness of less educated may impair the ability to use available health care services. Also, differences in the lifestyle contributed in widening the gap in health and mortality between educational groups. After the political change (started in 1989) accompanied by transformation toward market economy, better-educated people have been less likely to be unemployed and were better able to face economic hardship. They also have had higher income and more fulfilling and rewarding jobs than less educated individuals. All these facts imply that educational attainment (besides other factors) has played an important role for survival in any society, regardless of living under former socialism, capitalism, or new market economy. Increasing the amount of schooling can lower total level of mortality by two ways: (a) increasing share of highly educated people (with lower mortality) will impact total mortality level as structural effect and (b) faster decrease of death rates among higher educated adults will act as intensity effect. Therefore, in the next part, we model such situations in order to estimate the effects of changing population structure and mortality rates by education toward higher degrees.

4. Data and methods

The data on population structures by gender, age, and education come from the Population and Housing Census conducted in March 2011 (midnight from March 25 to 26th 2011) in the Czech Republic. The population counts were adjusted for the date of January 1, 2011 (by subtracting deaths between January 1 and March 25). The modified census counts were used as the denominator (mid-year population of the period 2009–2012) for mortality rates. Data on the number of deceased people according to gender, age, and education were derived from death certificates and served as the numerator for the mortality rates. Both data files (populations and deaths) were not linked because according to the Czech law, personal IDs had to be deleted after cleaning the raw census data.

The study focuses on the age group between 30 and 79 years. As a mortality indicator, it uses the temporary life expectancy between the exact ages 30 and 80. The age interval was chosen because educational attainment does not change almost at all after the age of 30, the death counts beyond the age of 80 are less frequent, and the information on education might be less reliable. In addition, age-specific mortality rates by education at age 80 and older converge.

Temporary life expectancy (life expectancy between two specific ages) measures the average number of years that a group of persons alive at exact age x will live from age x to $x + i$ years [33]

$$_ie_x = \frac{T_x - T_{x+i}}{l_x} \quad (1)$$

$_ie_x$ is the temporary life expectancy between exact ages x and $x + i$; T_x is the total number of person-years lived between exact ages x and $x + i$; and l_x is number surviving to the beginning of age interval x.

The data on population and deaths are classified into four educational attainment categories. This classification has been in use in the Czech Republic since the WWII: (1) less than high school degree is indicated as basic. It takes 9 years usually from the ages of 6 to 15 and consists of a primary and lower secondary stage, where the primary stage encompasses grades 1–5, whereas the lower secondary stage has grades 6–9 (**Table 1**). (2) Upper secondary education termed vocational (apprenticeships or training for skilled occupation) is generally 4 years in length (grades 10–13), and the certificate is not applicable for entering tertiary education. (3) Upper secondary general education (frequently from the age 15 with the usual length of 4 years), called secondary (grammar or high school resulting in a "Maturita" certificate), allows the entrance to the tertiary education. Tertiary or university education includes all studies following the completion of upper secondary education with a successful final examination and obtaining the Maturita certificate.

Three scenarios will be presented. The first one reflects the real situation, and the next two scenarios simulate the shifts toward a higher education: (a) population structure by sex, age and education will remain the same as from the census 2011 as well as mortality rates from 2009 to 2012 will not be changed (reference scenario); (b) change in population structure by education; 60% of males having the basic education will move into the next higher category (vocational) and 60% of women with basic and vocational education will move into the secondary education (it is because the difference in mortality between females with basic and vocational education is negligible); (c) change in death rates; sex age education-specific mortality rates will be shifted upwards by one level (basic = vocational, vocational = secondary, secondary = university, new university = 0.80*university).

Level of education	Educational attainment (ISCED 97)	Educational attainment (ISCED 2011)
Basic	ISCED 2	ISCED 2 and lower
Vocational	ISCED 3C	ISCED 35
Secondary	ISCED 3A	ISCED 34
University	ISCED 5A and higher	ISCED 64 and higher

Table 1. Classification of educational attainment in the Czech Republic based on ISCED codes.

5. Descriptive results

For the first introduction of the situation in mortality according to education attainment, the age-specific mortality rates were calculated, separately for each education level defined according to the ISCED levels (**Table 1**).

From the age-specific mortality rates, several the most important basic features are visible (**Figure 3a** and **b**). The first is a higher overall level of mortality for males—it holds for all of the education levels. The second observable feature in **Figure 3a** is the regular gradient of mortality levels according to education for males. In the case of males, the highest level of mortality is tied with the lowest level of education and vice versa.

The third feature observable in **Figure 3b** is the irregular gradient of mortality levels according to the education of females. This anomaly refers to the lowest education levels—basic and vocational. In particular, at higher ages (above 45), the level of mortality of females with basic education is lower in comparison with females with vocational education. There could be long discussions about the reasons for this anomaly; however, in general, it is assumed that this specificity could be tied to worse working conditions of females with vocational education in comparison with their less educated counterparts. Those females (with vocational education) worked more often manually in physically demanding jobs, in factories with substandard working conditions. On the other side, females with basic education worked more often in better conditions—as housewives, cleaners, etc.

Because the main goal of the study is to model possible changes of the education structure and their impact for the mortality changes, it is necessary to describe briefly the initial education structure of the population. The population structure by gender, age, and education attainment from the 2011 population census is shown in **Figure 4**. From the

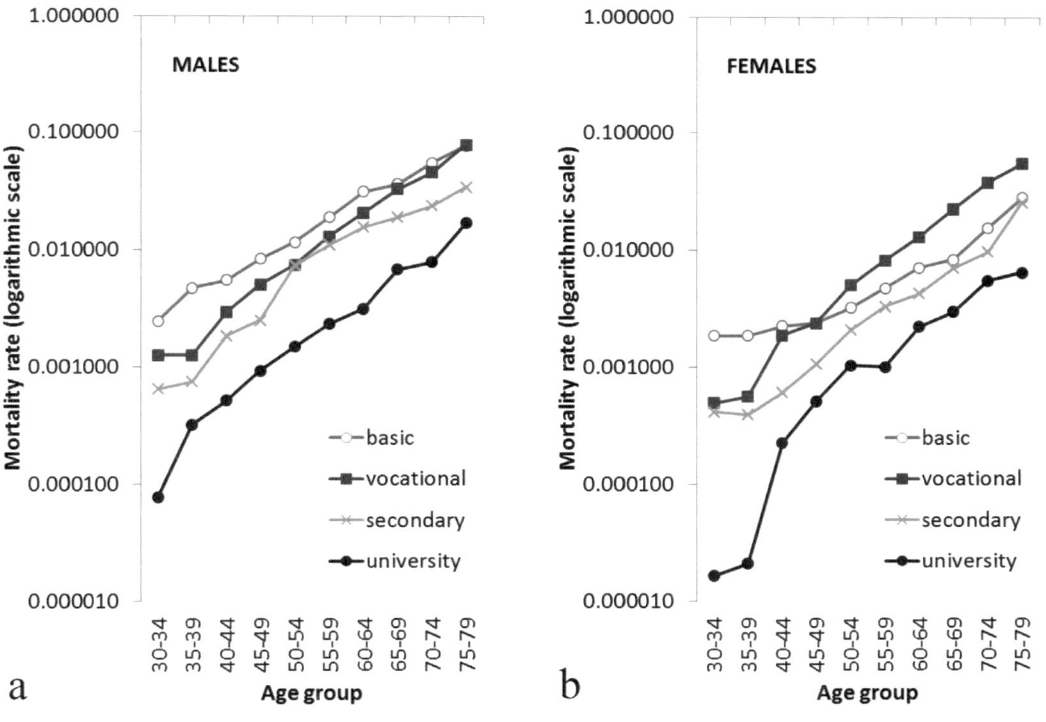

Figure 3. a) Czech Republic, age-specific mortality rates, years 2009–2012, males. b) Czech Republic, age-specific mortality rates, years 2009–2012, females.

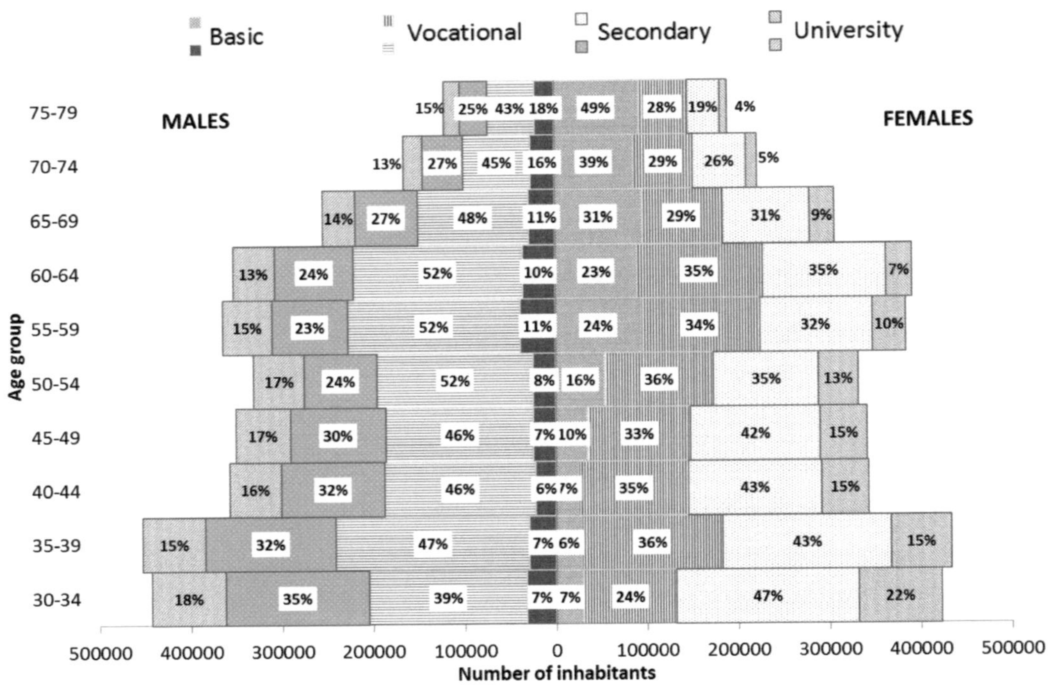

Figure 4. Czech Republic, population structure by gender, age, and education from the census 2011, ages 30–79 years.

population pyramid, many important differences could be pointed out. There is a clear increase in the proportion of the population with tertiary education with decreasing age. In the youngest age groups, the proportion of tertiary educated reached 22% for females and 18% for males. On the other side, with increasing age, the proportion of the population with only basic education rises, especially for females. At the highest age group (75–79 years), almost 50% of females had only basic education. In the case of males, the proportion was significantly lower—less than 20% at the oldest age groups and around 10% for the middle ages, and for the youngest age groups, the proportion was even lower. The most common education level for males is the vocational one (almost 50% share).

6. Model scenarios: shifting population or death rates by education

As was described in previous parts of the chapter, mortality in the Czech Republic is significantly different according to various levels of education. The aim of the following analysis was to transform the possible future changes of the education population structure or mortality rates into potential changes in temporary life expectancy. There are three different model scenarios defined with the purpose to illustrate the theoretically possible impacts on overall mortality caused by the changes in the education structure.

6.1. Scenario 1

The first model scenario could be indicated as a reference model. In this model, we suppose the education, gender, and age structures to remain unchanged. The population structure by education, gender, and age is that from the census 2011 (adjusted for January 1, 2011) and deaths rates those observed in the period 2009–2012. The population structure is graphically expressed by the population pyramid in **Figure 4** and mortality rates by education in **Figure 3a** and **b**.

The education structure from the 2011 census is characterized by a large proportion of people with only basic education at higher ages, especially for females. For males at the highest age groups, the proportion of basic education was only around 18% (in comparison to the proportion for females at the highest ages, which was almost 50%). At the youngest ages, the proportion of people with basic education decreased to only 7% for both the sexes. The largest proportion of males reached the vocational education (40–50% and this proportion is nearly invariant also at lower ages, except the youngest age group). For females, the vocational education was the second of importance at ages 65 and older. Women aged 30–49 most frequently had the secondary education. Moreover, for females, the proportion of basic education rapidly decreased from the highest age groups to the youngest ones and the proportion of secondary and university graduates increased with decreasing age. For males, almost the same trends can be depicted (see **Figure 4**).

6.2. Scenario 2

The second model scenario is characterized by only changes among people with the lowest levels of education. In this scenario, we suppose that 60% of males with only basic education will be moved into the higher category—vocational education. This assumption, in fact, reflects the decrease in the proportion of basic education with decreasing age as well as the high importance of vocational education among males.

For females, we suppose that 60% of females with basic and vocational education will move into the secondary education. Also, in this case, the reason for this assumption could be found in the decrease of the proportion of basic education with decreasing age and moreover the significant increase of the proportion of females with secondary education.

The modeled education structure corresponding with the Scenario 2 is illustrated by the population pyramid in **Figure 5**. According to this model scenario, the proportion of basic education nearly diminishes. On the other side, the proportion of vocational education for males would significantly increase together with the share of secondary education for females would significantly increase. It could be hypothesized that especially for females, this shift in educational structure could have a significant effect on the overall mortality level because the mortality rates of secondary education are visibly lower in comparison to basic and vocational education (see **Figure 3b**). Also in case of males, the effect of modeled changes in education attainment could be expected in order to lower overall mortality, however, not as significant as for females because the modeled change affects only the proportion of basic education which was low already in the real population (see the model Scenario 1).

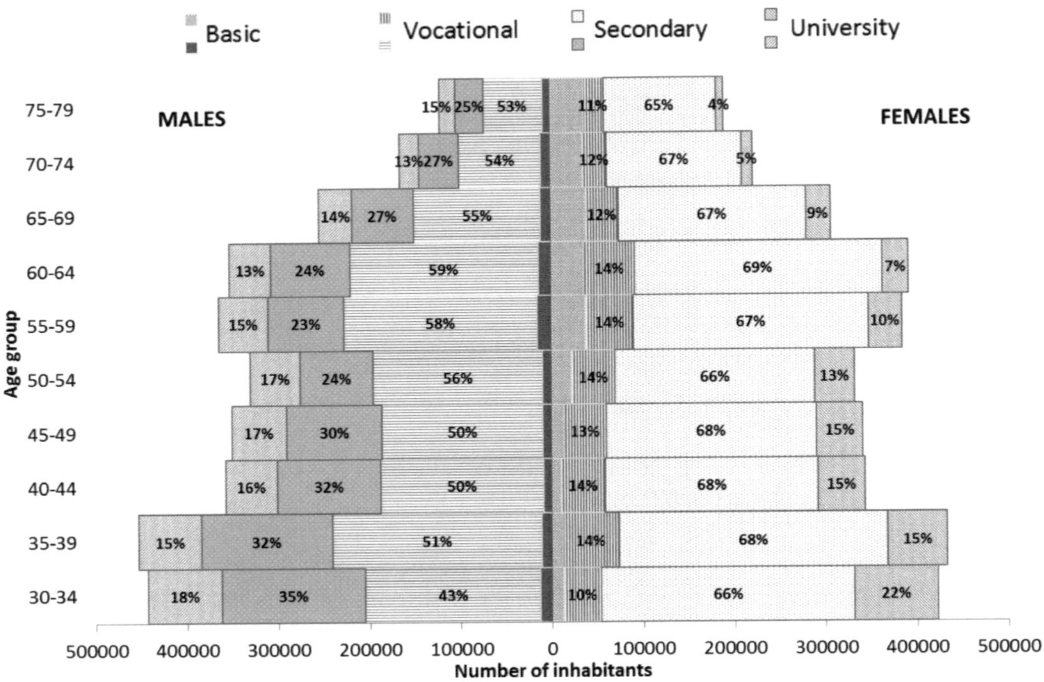

Figure 5. Population structure by gender, age, and education in the model Scenario 2, population aged 30–79 years.

6.3. Scenario 3

The last model scenario modifies all death rates by education while preserving population structure by education. In this model, we suppose shifts in sex age education-specific mortality rates upwards by one level (basic = vocational, vocational = secondary, secondary = university, new university = 0.80*university). The assumptions of this scenario are consistent with recent rapid changes in the educational structure of the Czech Republic, with a significant shift toward higher education levels. The proposed changes are supposed to impact overall mortality, above all in the case of males. The modeled shift according to this third scenario would lead to significant male mortality improvements due to their clear education gradient. The effect of change could be rather contradictory for females because women with vocational education experience slightly higher mortality compared to those with basic attainment (the above-mentioned anomaly in female mortality gradient by education, see **Figure 3b**). The shift from vocational education to secondary as well as changes connected with shifts toward university education would lower mortality levels for both genders.

7. Impact of education shifts on temporary life expectancy

The above-defined model scenarios of education shifts were further applied when calculating temporary life expectancies. Temporary life expectancies between exact ages 30 and 80 according to education attainment and based on Scenario 1 (no shifts) are presented in **Figure 6**.

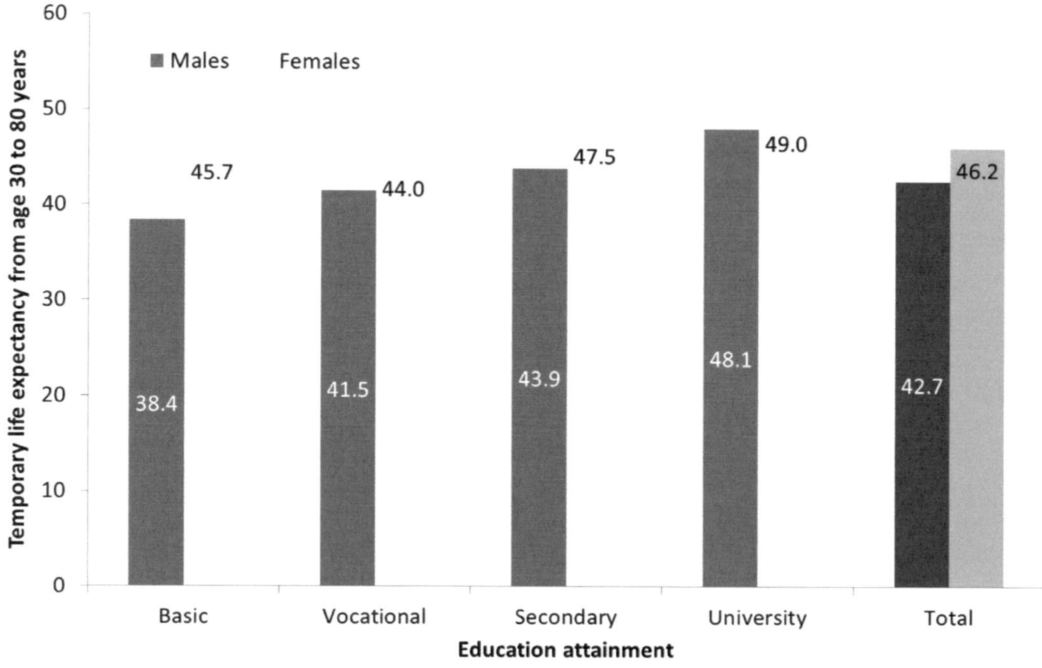

Figure 6. Temporary life expectancy for males and females between ages 30 and 80, Scenario 1, Scenario 2, Scenario 2 modified, and Scenario 3.

The most significant differences between males and females are visible for the basic level of education—for males this level of education is clearly the less favorable (**Figure 6**). However, females with basic education show longer temporary life expectancy (45.7 years) compared to those having a vocational degree (44.0 years). The total temporary life expectancy from age 30 to 80 was 42.7 years for males and 46.2 years for females.

According to the Scenario 2, the population of the least educated (basic) males was reduced and the majority of them (60%) moved into the higher educated (vocational) group. About 60% of females with basic and vocational education was moved into the secondary education. The effect of lowering mortality, based on temporary life expectancy, was significant only for females due to a large decrease in the share of women with basic and vocational education moved into the secondary degree. Consequently, the total female temporary life expectancy increased (47.1–46.2 = 0.9) by almost a year (**Figures 6** and **7**). For males, the effect of the shift in educational population structure was negligible—the temporary life expectancy increased by only 0.1 years (42.8–42.7 = 0.1). The reasons were already stated, the proposed change in population educational structure (from basic into vocational) involved only a relatively small group of males. Therefore, a modified Scenario 2 was elaborated for males.

Modification of the Scenario 2 only consists in another shifting of the male population structure by education (females movement is the same as in Scenario 2). According to the modified Scenario 2, 60% of males with vocational education was moved toward secondary education (60% with basic

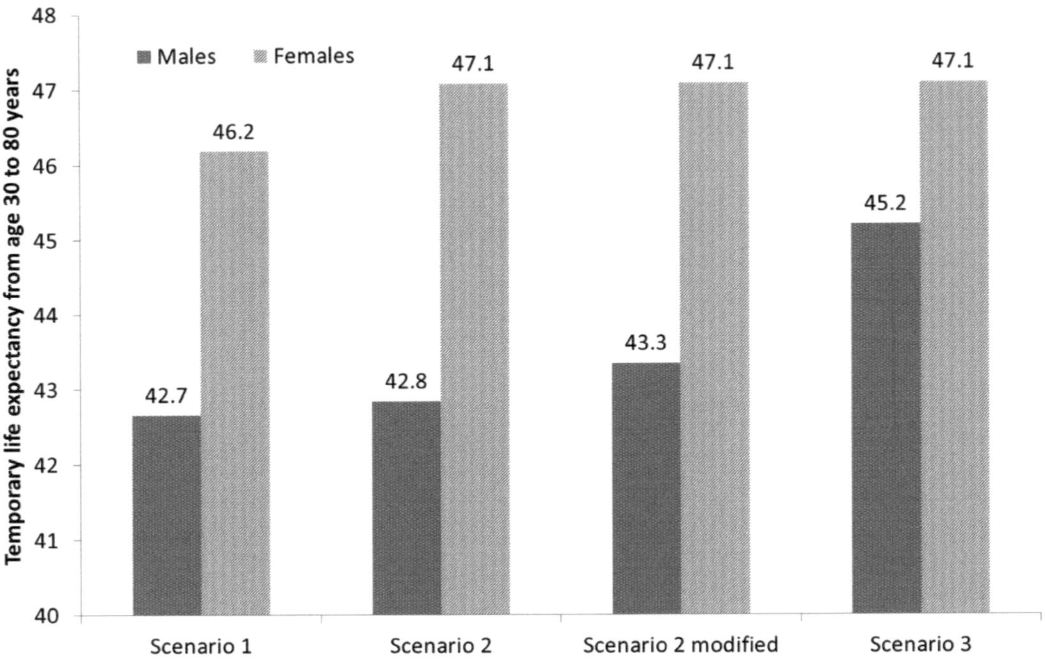

Figure 7. Temporary life expectancy between ages 30 and 80 for males and females, Scenarios 1, 2 (without and with modification), and 3.

education moved into vocational). This assumption is in line with the general tendency in the educational structure of the Czech population over time, where secondary education is expanding for males. Because the vocational education group of males is relatively large, we can expect that the resulting effect on temporary life expectancy will be higher than in the Scenario 2 (without modification). Of course, for females, the results will be the same based on Scenario 2 or Scenario 2 modified. The results are shown in **Figure 7**. As it was assumed, the shift of high proportion of the male population with vocational education toward secondary (Scenario 2 modified) had a more significant impact on the rise of the temporary life expectancy between ages 30 and 80—it increased from the initial value of 42.7 to 43.3 years. Based on the Scenario 2 or Scenario 2 modified, it is possible to expect a future growth of the life expectancy caused (among others) by the ongoing changes of population education structure. The improving education structure of the population could lead to an increase in the temporary life expectancy between ages 30 and 80 by nearly a year.

The results based on the Scenario 3 (shifting death rates toward higher education category) were to be the most optimistic ones, especially for males. In the case of females, lower mortality of women with basic education compared to their vocational counterparts can produce a contradictory effect and thus reduce the growth of temporary life expectancy. The general shift in the education structure toward higher levels is likely and is consistent with the ongoing education development in the Czech Republic. From the results (see **Figure 7**), it is seen that initial hypotheses were correct. The estimated outputs (hypothetical temporary life expectancies) are clearly more favorable in case of males (gain of

45.2–42.7 = 2.5 years) in comparison with females (gain of 47.1–46.2 = 0.9 years). The male advantage is closely connected to the shifts of high mortality education categories (basic or vocational) toward much favorable survival experienced by men having a secondary or a university degree. Females show a less pronounced gradient in mortality by education, and therefore, mortality reduction is rather modest. Such a trend is in line with findings in other countries [9, 15].

The complete disappearance of the most unfavorable group of males (with only basic education) or females having a basic or vocational education is unlikely. Therefore, future mortality decline will be primarily driven by lowering sex age education-specific mortality rates. It is the field of health and social policies on one side and personal responsibility for one's own health and for successfully functioning in a society on the other side.

8. Conclusion

In recent years, the population of the Czech Republic experienced two important phenomena: increase in the share of higher educated people and a significant decline in mortality at adult ages. The impact of changing education structure (in population as well as in rates) can be especially influential due to large disparities in survival according to educational attainment in the Czech Republic. Because these differences are among the largest in Europe, further studies of related factors are needed. Scientific understanding of determinants of educational differences of adult mortality has increased substantially over the past few decades in developed countries. Some striking phenomena have been identified: (a) educational differences in mortality rates have widened over the past several decades despite a dramatic progression of life expectancy, (b) mortality inequalities by education among women are rising over time ant thus approaching male patterns, and (c) regional differences in mortality by education are more pronounced when comparing with national patterns.

In our contribution, the main goal was to model the potential development in mortality under the various conditions addressing the education shift in the society. Based on the scenarios and their assumptions, the changes in temporary life expectancy between ages 30 and 80 were estimated. The results have shown that a decrease of the proportion of the population with the lowest education would lead to only a small increase in temporary life expectancy. On the other hand, decreasing education specific death rates have a larger impact on aggregate mortality indicators. However, it has to be kept in mind that even a small sub-group of the population matters and is worth considering when looking at the overall mortality level.

Acknowledgements

The study was supported by the Czech Science Foundation, project No. P404-12-0883.

Author details

Jitka Rychtaříková* and Klára Hulíková Tesárková

*Address all correspondence to: rychta@natur.cuni.cz

Department of Demography and Geodemography, Faculty of Science, Charles University, Prague, Czech Republic

References

[1] Kitagawa E, Hauser P. Differential mortality in the United States: A study in socioeconomic epidemiology. Cambridge: Harvard University Press; 1973. p. 288

[2] Department of Health and Social Security, editors. The Black Report 1980. Inequalities in Health. Report of a Research Working Group. DHSS ed. London: Socialist Health Association; 1980

[3] Hoffmann R. Do socioeconomic mortality differences decrease with rising age? Demographic Research. 2005;**13**(2):35-62. DOI: 10.4054/DemRes.2005.13.2

[4] Kibele EUB, Jasilionis D, Shkolnikov VM. Widening socioeconomic differences in mortality among men aged 65 years and older in Germany. Journal of Epidemiology & Community Health. 2013;**67**(5):453-457. DOI: 10.1136/jech-2012-201761

[5] Lantz PM, House JS, Lepkowski JM, Williams DR, Mero RP, Chen J. Socioeconomic Factors, Health Behaviors, and Mortality. JAMA. 1998;**279**(21):1703-1708. DOI: 10.1001/jama.279.21.1703

[6] Mackenbach JP, Kunst AE, Groenhof F, Borgan JK, Costa G, Faggiano F, et al. Socioeconomic inequalities in mortality among women and among men: An international study. American Journal of Public Health. 1999;**89**(12):1800-1806. DOI: 10.2105/AJPH.89.12.1800

[7] Mustard CA, Etches J. Gender differences in socioeconomic inequality in mortality. Journal of Epidemiology & Community Health. 2003;**57**(12):974-980. DOI: 10.1136/jech.57.12.974

[8] Vandenheede H, Vikhirev O, Pikhart H, Kubinova R, Malyutina S, Pajak A, et al. Socioeconomic inequalities in all-cause mortality in the Czech Republic, Russia, Poland and Lithuania in the 2000s: Findings from the HAPIEE Study. Journal of Epidemiology & Community Health. 2014;**68**(4):297-303. DOI: 10.1136/jech-2013-203057

[9] Karas Montez J, Zajacova A. Trends in mortality risk by education level and cause of death among US white women from 1986 to 2006. American Journal of Public Health. 2013;**103**(3):473-479. DOI: 10.2105/AJPH.2012.301128

[10] Kunst AE, Bos V, Andersen O, Cardano M, Costa G, Harding S, et al. Monitoring of trends in socioeconomic inequalities in mortality: Experiences from a European project. Demographic Research, Special collection. 2004;**2**(9):229-254. DOI: 10.4054/DemRes.2004.S2.9

[11] Mackenbach JP, Bakker MJ. Tackling socioeconomic inequalities in health: analysis of European experiences. The Lancet. 2003;**362**(9393):1409-1414. DOI: 10.1016/S0140-6736(03)14639-9

[12] Masters RK, Hummer RA, Powersb DA. Educational differences in U.S. adult mortality: A cohort perspective. American Sociological Review. 2012;**77**(4):548-572. DOI: 10.1177/0003122412451019

[13] Elo IT, Preston S. Educational differentials in mortality: United States. Social Science & Medicine. 1996;**42**(1):47-57. DOI: 10.1016/0277-9536(95)00062-3

[14] Brown DC, Hayward MD, Karas Montez J, Hummer RA, Chiu CT, Hidajat MM. The significance of education for mortality compression. Demography. 2012;**49**(3):819-840. DOI: 10.1007/s13524-012-0104-1

[15] Hummer RA, Hernandez EM. The effect of educational attainment on adult mortality in the United States. Population Bulletin. 2013;**68**(1):1-16

[16] Christenson BA, Johnson NE. Educational inequality in adult mortality: An assessment with death certificate data from Michigan. Demography. 1995;**32**(2):215-229. DOI: 10.2307/2061741

[17] Klotz J, Doblhammer G. Trends in educational mortality differentials in Austria between 1981/82 and 2001/2002. Demographic Research. 2008;**19**(2):1759-1780. DOI: 10.4054/DemRes.2008.19.51

[18] van Raalte AA, Kunst AE, Deboosere P, Leinsalu M, Lundberg O, Martikainen P, et al. More variation in lifespan in lower educated. International Journal of Epidemiology. 2011;**40**(6):1703-1714. DOI: 10.1093/ije/dyr146

[19] Zajacova A, Hummer RA. Gender differences in education effects on all-cause mortality for white and black adults in the United States. Social Science & Medecine. 2009;**69**(4):529-537. DOI: 10.1016/j.socscimed.2009.06.028

[20] Bobak M, Marmot M. East-West mortality divide and its potential explanations: Proposed research agenda. British Medical Journal, International edition. 1996;**312**(7028):421-425. DOI: 10.3109/13814789609161649

[21] Woolf SH, Johnson RE, Phillips RL, Philipsen M. Giving everyone the health of the educated: An examination of whether social change would save. American Journal of Public Health. 2007;**97**(4):679-683. DOI: 10.2105/AJPH.2005.084848

[22] Arias E, Heron M, Xu JQ, Division of Vital Statistics. National vital statistics reports. United States Life Tables, 2012. 2016;**65**(8):1-68

[23] Czech Statistical Office. 2016. https://www.czso.cz/csu/czso/life_Tables

[24] Espérance de vie. INED. 2016. http://www.ined.fr/fr/tout-savoir-population/chiffres/france/mortalite-cause-deces/esperance-vie/

[25] Pison G. Population trends in the United States and Europe: Similarities and differences. Population & Societies. 2008;**446**(June):1-4

[26] Belloni A, Sassi. Health-care expenditure and health policy in the USA versus other high-spending OECD. The Lancet. 2014;**384**(9937):83-92. DOI: 10.1016/S0140-6736(14)61032-1

[27] Jaffe H, Frieden T. Improving health in the USA: Progress and challenges. The Lancet. 2014;**384**(9937):3-4. DOI: 10.1016/S0140-6736(14)61032-1

[28] Rychtaříková J. Education and survival in the Czech Republic. Acta Universitatis Carolinae Geographica. 2005;**40**(1-2):123-137

[29] Rychtaříková J, Vallin J, Meslé F. Comparative study of mortality trends in France and the Czech Republic since 1950. Population. English Selection. 1989;**44**(1):291-321

[30] Rychtaříková J. The case of the Czech Republic: Determinants of the recent favourable turnover in mortality. Demographic Research, Special Collection. 2004;**2**(5):105-138. DOI: 10.4054/DemRes.2004.S2.5

[31] Central and Eastern Europe in transition public policy and social conditions. Crisis in mortality, health and nutrition. Economies in Transition Studies. Regional Monitoring Report. 1994;(**2**):110

[32] Beckett M. Converging health inequalities in later life—An artifact of mortality selection?. Journal of Health & Social Behavior. 2000;**41**(1):106-119

[33] Arriaga EE. Measuring and explaining the change in life expectancies. Demography. 1984;**21**(1):106-119